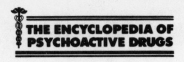

THE ENCYCLOPEDIA OF PSYCHOACTIVE DRUGS

IN 25 VOLUMES
Each title on a specific drug or drug-related problem

BARBITURATES

THE ENCYCLOPEDIA OF PSYCHOACTIVE DRUGS

BARBITURATES

Sleeping Potion or Intoxicant?

JACK E. HENNINGFIELD, Ph.D.

Johns Hopkins University School of Medicine

NANCY ALMAND ATOR, Ph.D.

Johns Hopkins University School of Medicine

1986
CHELSEA HOUSE PUBLISHERS
NEW YORK
NEW HAVEN   PHILADELPHIA

COVER: René Magritte, *Les Rêveries du Promeneur Solitaire.* Estate of René Magritte. Copyright © 1986.

SENIOR EDITOR: William P. Hansen
PROJECT EDITOR: Jane Larkin Crain
ASSISTANT EDITOR: Paula Edelson
EDITORIAL COORDINATOR: Karyn Gullen Browne
EDITORIAL STAFF: Jeff Freiert
        Perry Scott King
        Kathleen McDermott
        Alma Rodriguez-Sokol
ART DIRECTOR: Susan Lusk
ART COORDINATOR: Carol McDougall
LAYOUT: Noreen M. Lamb
ART ASSISTANT: Victoria Tomaselli
PICTURE RESEARCH: Elizabeth Terhune, Diane Moroff

ACKNOWLEDGMENTS: Pp. 34–38: American Medical Association. *Archives of Neurology and Psychiatry*, July, 1950, pp. 1–28. H. Isbell, et al. P. 55: Dyker, M.W., Kooser, J.A., Haraszti, J.S., and Davis, J.M. Clinical usefulness of sodium amobarbital interviewing. *Archives of General Psychiatry* 1979, vol. 36, pp. 789–794. Pp. 66–67: Kessell, N. "Psychiatric Aspects of Acute Barbiturate Poisoning," from *Acute Barbiturate Poisoning*, H. Matthew, editor. Amsterdam: Excerpta Medica, 1971, pp. 270–290.

Library of Congress Cataloging in Publication Data
Henningfield, Jack E.
    Barbiturates: sleeping potion or intoxicant?
    (The Encyclopedia of psychoactive drugs)
    Bibliography: p.
    Includes index.
    Summary: Discusses the effects, side effects, and dangers of barbiturate use and abuse.
    1. Barbiturates—Juvenile literature.
2. Barbiturates—Toxicology—Juvenile literature.
[1. Barbiturates. 2. Drugs. 3. Drug abuse]
I. Ator, Nancy Almand. II. Title. III. Series.
RM325.H46   1986   615'.78   85-17432
ISBN 0-87754-768-8

Chelsea House Publishers
Harold Steinberg, Chairman & Publisher
Susan Lusk, Vice President
A Division of Chelsea House Educational Communications, Inc.

133 Christopher Street, New York, NY 10014

345 Whitney Avenue, New Haven, CT 05510

5014 West Chester Pike, Edgemont, PA 19028

CONTENTS

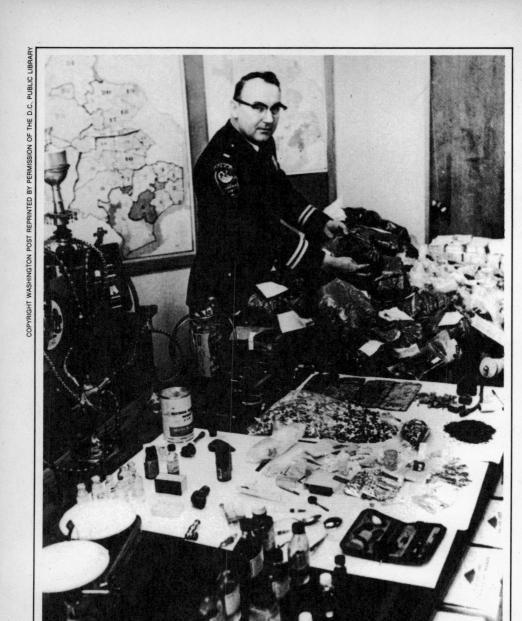

A police officer surveys a small fortune of confiscated drugs. Although the abuse of barbiturates is not particularly widespread today, it reached epidemic proportions during the 1950s and 1960s.

FOREWORD

In the Mainstream of American Life

The rapid growth of drug use and abuse is one of the most dramatic changes in the fabric of American society in the last 20 years. The United States has the highest level of psychoactive drug use of any industrialized society. It is 10 to 30 times greater than it was 20 years ago.

According to a recent Gallup poll, young people consider drugs the leading problem that they face. One of the legacies of the social upheaval of the 1960s is that psychoactive drugs have become part of the mainstream of American life. Schools, homes, and communities cannot be "drug proofed." There is a demand for drugs—and the supply is plentiful. Social norms have changed and drugs are not only available—they are everywhere.

Almost all drug use begins in the preteen and teenage years. These years are few in the total life cycle, but critical in the maturation process. During these years adolescents face the difficult tasks of discovering their identity, clarifying their sexual roles, asserting their independence, learning to cope with authority, and searching for goals that will give their lives meaning. During this intense period of growth, conflict is inevitable and the temptation to use drugs is great. Drugs are readily available, adolescents are curious and vulnerable, there is peer pressure to experiment, and there is the temptation to escape from conflicts.

No matter what their age or socioeconomic status, no group is immune to the allure and effects of psychoactive drugs. The U.S. Surgeon General's report, "Healthy People," indicates that 30% of all deaths in the United States

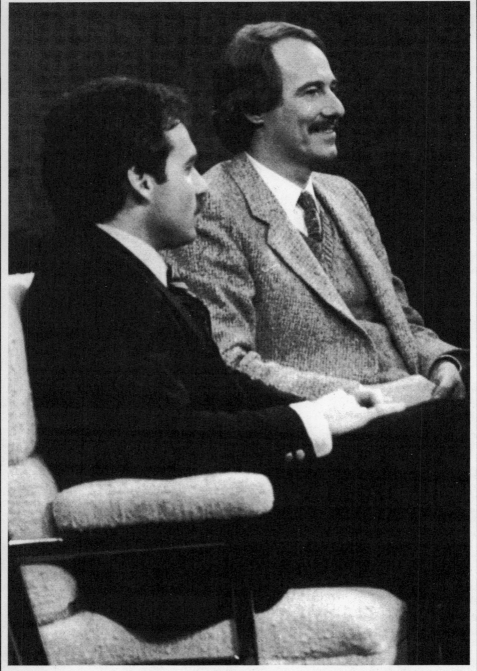

Singer John Phillips (right) discusses his former drug problem with Dr. Mark S. Gold, who founded the Cocaine Hotline. Phillips, who was addicted to barbiturates, is now involved with anti-drug campaigns.

are premature because of alcohol and tobacco use. However, the most shocking development in this report is that mortality in the age group between 15 and 24 has increased since 1960 despite the fact that death rates for all other age groups have declined in the 20th century. Accidents, suicides, and homicides are the leading cause of death in young people 15 to 24 years of age. In many cases the deaths are directly related to drug use.

THE ENCYCLOPEDIA OF PSYCHOACTIVE DRUGS answers the questions that young people are likely to ask about drugs, as well as those they might not think to ask, but should. Topics include: what it means to be intoxicated; how drugs affect mood; why people take drugs; who takes them; when they take them; and how much they take. They will learn what happens to a drug when it enters the body. They will learn what it means to get "hooked" and how it happens. They will learn how drugs affect their driving, their schoolwork, and those around them—their peers, their family, their friends, and their employers. They will learn what the signs are that indicate that a friend or a family member may have a drug problem and to identify four stages leading from drug use to drug abuse. Myths about drugs are dispelled.

National surveys indicate that students are eager for information about drugs and that they respond to it. Students not only need information about drugs—they want information. How they get it often proves crucial. Providing young people with accurate knowledge about drugs is one of the most critical aspects.

THE ENCYCLOPEDIA OF PSYCHOACTIVE DRUGS synthesizes the wealth of new information in this field and demystifies this complex and important subject. Each volume in the series is written by an expert in the field. Handsomely illustrated, this multi-volume series is geared for teenage readers. Young people will read these books, share them, talk about them, and make more informed decisions because of them.

Miriam Cohen, Ph.D.
Contributing Editor

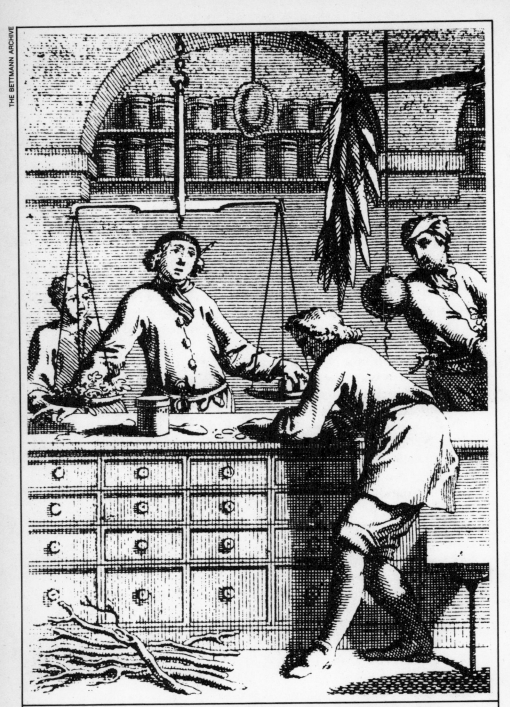

A 17th-century drawing of a physician prescribing medicinal plants.
Modern doctors employ many synthetic drugs for the treatment of disease.
Barbiturates are among the most widely used of these compounds.

INTRODUCTION

The Gift of Wizardry
Use and Abuse

JACK H. MENDELSON, M.D.

NANCY K. MELLO, PH.D.

Alcohol and Drug Abuse Research Center
Harvard Medical School—McLean Hospital

Dorothy to the Wizard:

"I think you are a very bad man," said Dorothy.
"Oh, no, my dear; I'm really a very good man; but I'm a very bad Wizard."

—from THE WIZARD OF OZ

Man is endowed with the gift of wizardry, a talent for discovery and invention. The discovery and invention of substances that change the way we feel and behave are among man's special accomplishments, and like so many other products of our wizardry, these substances have the capacity to harm as well as to help. The substance itself is neutral, an intricate molecular structure. Yet, "too much" can be sickening, even deadly. It is man who decides how each substance is used, and it is man's beliefs and perceptions that give this neutral substance the attributes to heal or destroy.

Consider alcohol—available to all and yet regarded with intense ambivalence from biblical times to the present day. The use of alcoholic beverages dates back to our earliest ancestors. Alcohol use and misuse became associated with the worship of gods and demons. One of the most powerful Greek gods was Dionysus, lord of fruitfulness and god of wine. The Romans adopted Dionysus but changed his name to Bacchus. Festivals and holidays associated with Bacchus celebrated the harvest and the origins of life. Time has blurred the images of the Bacchanalian festival, but the theme of drunkenness as a major part of celebration has survived the pagan gods and remains a familiar part of modern society.

The term "Bacchanalian festival" conveys a more appealing image than "drunken orgy" or "pot party," but whatever the label, some of the celebrants will inevitably start up the "high" escalator to the next plateau. Once there, the de-escalation is difficult for many.

According to reliable estimates, one out of every ten Americans develops a serious alcohol-related problem sometime in his or her lifetime. In addition, automobile accidents caused by drunken drivers claim the lives of tens of thousands every year. Many of the victims are gifted young people, just starting out in adult life. Hospital emergency rooms abound with patients seeking help for alcohol-related injuries.

Who is to blame? Can we blame the many manufacturers who produce such an amazing variety of alcoholic beverages? Should we blame the educators who fail to explain the perils of intoxication, or so exaggerate the dangers of drinking that no one could possibly believe them? Are friends to blame—those peers who urge others to "drink more and faster," or the macho types who stress the importance of being able to "hold your liquor"? Casting blame, however, is hardly constructive, and pointing the finger is a fruitless way to deal with problems. Alcoholism and drug abuse have few culprits but many victims. Accountability begins with each of us, every time we choose to use or to misuse an intoxicating substance.

It is ironic that some of man's earliest medicines, derived from natural plant products, are used today to poison and to intoxicate. Relief from pain and suffering is one of society's many continuing goals. Over 3,000 years ago, the Therapeutic Papyrus of Thebes, one of our earliest written records, gave instructions for the use of opium in the treatment of pain. Opium, in the form of its major derivative, morphine, remains one of the most powerful drugs we have for pain relief. But opium, morphine, and similar compounds, such as heroin, have also been used by many to induce changes in mood and feeling. Another example of man's misuse of a natural substance is the coca leaf, which for centuries was used by the Indians of Peru to reduce fatigue and hunger. Its modern derivative, cocaine, has important medical use as a local anesthetic. Unfortunately, its increasing abuse in the 1980s has reached epidemic proportions.

The purpose of this series is to provide information about the nature and behavioral effects of alcohol and drugs, and the probable consequences of their use. The information presented here (and in other books in this series) is based on many clinical and laboratory studies and observations by people from diverse walks of life.

Over the centuries, novelists, poets, and dramatists have provided us with many insights into the beneficial and problematic aspects of alcohol and drug use. Physicians, lawyers, biologists, psychologists, and social scientists have contributed to a better understanding of the causes and consequences of using these substances. The authors in this series have attempted to gather and condense all the latest information about drug use and abuse. They have also described the sometimes wide gaps in our knowledge and have suggested some new ways to answer many difficult questions.

One such question, for example, is how do alcohol and drug problems get started? And what is the best way to treat them when they do? Not too many years ago, alcoholics and drug abusers were regarded as evil, immoral, or both. It is now recognized that these persons suffer from very complicated diseases involving complex biological, psychological, and social problems. To understand how the disease begins and progresses, it is necessary to understand the nature of the substance, the behavior and genetic makeup of the afflicted person, and the characteristics of the society or culture in which he lives.

The diagram below shows the interaction of these three factors. The arrows indicate that the substance not only affects the user personally, but the society as well. Society influences attitudes towards the substance, which in turn affect its availability. The substance's impact upon the society may support or discourage the use and abuse of that substance.

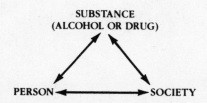

SUBSTANCE
(ALCOHOL OR DRUG)

PERSON ⟷ SOCIETY

Although many of the social environments we live in are very similar, some of the most subtle differences can strongly influence our thinking and behavior. Where we live, go to school and work, whom we discuss things with—all influence our opinions about drug use and misuse. Yet we also share certain commonly accepted beliefs that outweigh any differences in our attitudes. The authors in this series have tried to identify and discuss the central, most crucial issues concerning drug use and misuse.

Regrettably, man's wizardry in developing new substances in medical therapeutics has not always been paralleled by intelligent usage. Although we do know a great deal about the effects of alcohol and drugs, we have yet to learn how to impart that knowledge, especially to young adults.

Does it matter? What harm does it do to smoke a little pot or have a few beers? What is it like to be intoxicated? How long does it last? Will it make me feel really fine? Will it make me sick? What are the risks? These are but a few of the questions answered in this series, which, hopefully, will enable the reader to make wise decisions concerning the crucial issue of drugs.

Information sensibly acted upon can go a long way towards helping everyone develop his or her best self. As one keen and sensitive observer, Dr. Lewis Thomas, has said,

> *There is nothing at all absurd about the human condition. We matter. It seems to me a good guess, hazarded by a good many people who have thought about it, that we may be engaged in the formation of something like a mind for the life of this planet. If this is so, we are still at the most primitive stage, still fumbling with language and thinking, but infinitely capacitated for the future. Looked at this way, it is remarkable that we've come as far as we have in so short a period, really no time at all as geologists measure time. We are the newest, the youngest, and the brightest thing around.*

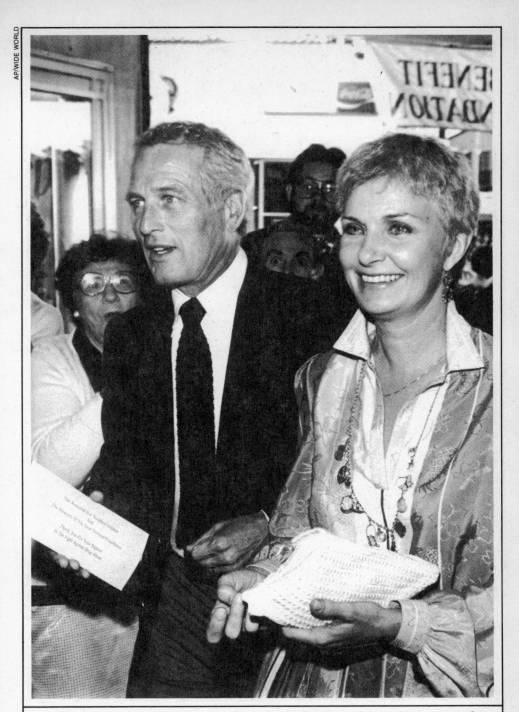

Paul Newman and Joanne Woodward at a function that raised money for the Scott Newman Foundation. Named after the couple's dead son, the organization runs drug-abuse prevention programs for children.

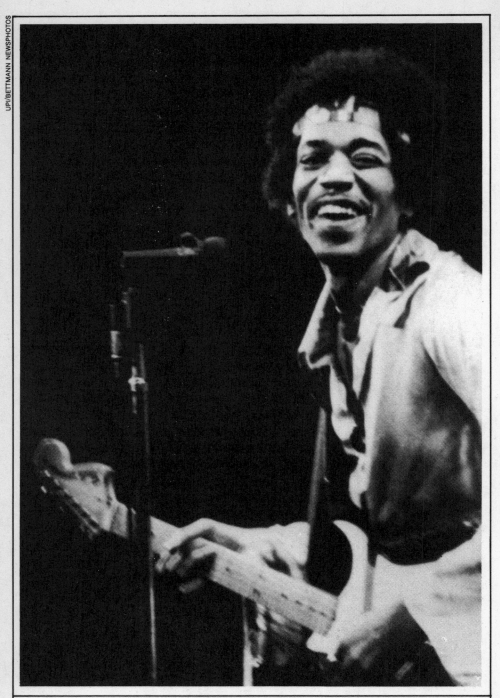

Jimi Hendrix, one of the most popular rock stars of the 1960s, died at the age of 28 when he choked on his own vomit after taking barbiturates, which slow the throat reflexes and depress respiration.

AUTHOR'S PREFACE

The discovery of barbiturates at the beginning of the 20th century marked a major advance in medicine. They provided relief for sufferers of two very common ailments—anxiety and insomnia.

One good measure of a drug is the degree to which it cures without producing negative side effects. Judged by this standard, barbiturates were far from perfect. All cases of anxiety were not eased, and in some cases the sleep they did produce was not refreshing. Furthermore, improper or too frequent use of the drug could lead to dependency. Overuse could lead to intoxication or even death. But for thousands of patients they were effective and certainly far more tolerable than any drugs previously used for similar purposes.

So what are barbiturates? How do they work? Are they still important to modern health care? Why do they produce dependence? Who is likely to become addicted to them and how can such people be treated? This book will explore these and related issues.

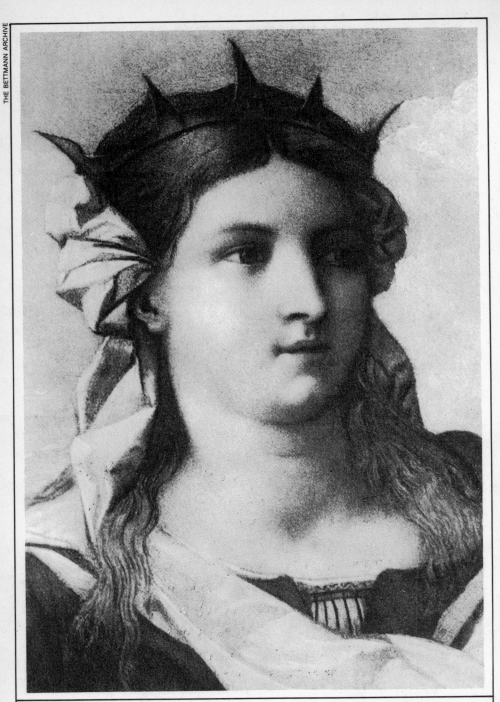

Because Adolph von Baeyer discovered a new chemical on the Feast Day of Saint Barbara (above), he combined the saint's name and the chemical name urea to form the word for his new find—barbiturates.

CHAPTER 1

WHAT ARE BARBITURATES?

*B*arbiturates are derived from barbituric acid, a chemical discovered in 1863 by a 29-year-old research assistant in a Belgian laboratory. The story has it that the researcher, Adolph von Baeyer, produced the acid from the condensation of malonic acid and urea and went to a local tavern to celebrate his discovery. There he found some army officers enjoying a celebration of their own to. mark the Day of St. Barbara, the patron saint of artillerymen and others who handle explosives. According to this story, von Baeyer combined the name of St. Barbara and the chemical name urea to form the name for his new discovery—barbiturates.

Forty years later, two German scientists, Emil Hermann Fischer and Joseph von Mering, used von Baeyer's acid to synthesize a new drug which they called barbital. It was marketed under the name Veronal and is still sold today.

Like many others before them, Fischer and von Mering had been looking for a drug that would combat the effects of anxiety and nervousness. Some success had been achieved with narcotics such as opium, codeine, and morphine. But their side effects, most notably the potential for addiction, made them unsuitable except in emergencies. Naturally occurring bromide salts had also been used to induce sleep, but prolonged use could lead to poisoning. Chloral hydrate and paraldehyde were also partially successful, but they tasted and smelled terrible and gave their users extremely bad breath.

Fischer and von Mering found that barbital was a useful hypnotic that could induce sleep in both humans and animals. And it was soon in widespread use. Almost a decade later, in 1912, a second barbiturate, phenobarbital, was introduced into medicine as a sedative-hypnotic, that is, a drug that induces relaxation, relief from anxiety, and sleep. It was sold under the brand name Luminal and, like Veronal, it too is still available.

Since that time, more than 2,000 similar chemicals have been developed, although only about 50 were actually marketed for public use in clinical medicine. They gave doctors unprecedented tools for treating sleep and anxiety disorders. They were relatively tasteless, odorless, and did not give the

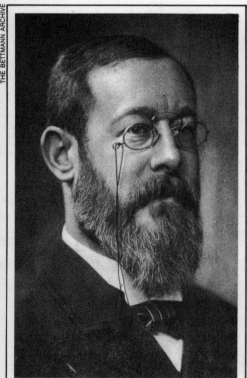
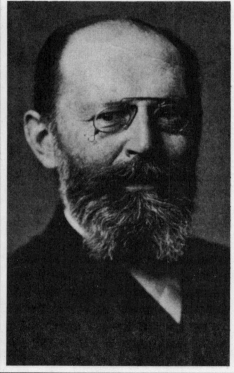

Joseph von Mering (left; 1849–1908) and Emil Fischer (1852–1919), two German scientists who in 1903 synthesized a new drug from barbituric acid. They called it barbital, and it was marketed under the name Veronal. Still available today, Veronal was found to be an effective sedative/hypnotic with, unfortunately, some significant side effects.

user bad breath. At the right dose level, they could enable the anxiety-stricken patient to function well socially, at home, and on the job. At higher dosages, some of the barbiturates produced speedy and satisfactory sleep.

Unfortunately, the profound complications associated with barbiturate use quickly became apparent. Soon after the drugs were introduced reports of fatal poisoning began to arise. And as the use of the drugs grew, so did the number of deaths associated with them, until in some countries they were the cause of more deaths than any other compound. For instance, during the mid-1950s, 70% of all admissions at the poison treatment center in Copenhagen, Denmark, were due to barbiturate overdose. In the 1960s the introduction of alternative compounds such as Valium and Librium resulted in a decline in barbiturate-related overdoses, but the danger is still substantial.

Depressants and Sedative-Hypnotics

The pharmacology of a drug refers to how it affects the functioning of organisms. Drugs that change a person's mood, feelings, or behavior generally work by affecting the central nervous system, or the brain. In this regard, barbiturates are classified as central nervous system depressants because their main effect is to depress or slow the activity of the central nervous system.

In clinical medicine, drugs are categorized by their usefulness. Thus, barbiturates are called sedative-hypnotics because their main effect is to calm, sedate, and produce drowsiness or sleep.

But both pharmacologists and clinical doctors agree on a classification system for how long the effects of a particular barbiturate will last. They are classified as short-acting (4 hours or less), intermediate-acting (4–6 hours), and long-acting (6 or more hours). There is also a special classification for ultra-short-acting barbiturates, which are usually given by intravenous injection and which may produce sedation before the injection is completed.

There are, however, shortcomings in classifying barbiturates by the duration of their actions. Experts agree that these time frames are approximations, and that duration of action can vary according to a number of different factors,

Table 1

Depressants' Duration of Action			
GENERIC NAME	TRADE OR BRAND NAME	DURATION OF ACTION*	RELATIVE ABUSE POTENTIAL
Barbiturates			
secobarbital	Seconal	short	high
pentobarbital sodium	Nembutal Sodium	short	high
talbutal	Lotusate	short	moderate
secobarbital and amobarbital	Tuinal	short-intermediate	high
butalbital	Sandoptal (in Fiorinal)	short-intermediate	moderate
amobarbital	Amytal	intermediate	high
butabarbital	Butisol	intermediate	moderate
phenobarbital	Luminal	long	low
Barbituratelike Substances			
methyprylon	Noludar	short	moderate
methaqualone	Quaalude	short	high
ethchlorvynol	Placidyl	short	low-moderate
ethinamate	Valmid	short	low
glutethimide	Doriden	intermediate	low-moderate
Benzodiazepines			
triazolam	Halcion	ultra-short	low
lorazepam	Ativan	short	low
flurazepam	Dalmane	short	low
diazepam	Valium	intermediate	low
oxazepam	Serax	long	low
chlordiazepoxide	Librium	long	low
Other Depressants			
chloral hydrate	Noctec	short	low
chloral betaine	Beta-Chlor	short	low
paraldehyde	Paral	short	low
meprobamate	Miltown, Equanil	intermediate	low

*Short-acting: 4 hours or less; intermediate-acting: 4–6 hours; long-acting: 6 or more hours.

including physiological differences among individual patients, the amount of the dose and the way in which it is administered. For example, a low dose of a long-acting barbiturate given intravenously will probably have a shorter effect than a larger dose of an intermediate-acting barbiturate taken orally. In general, it takes long-acting barbiturates relatively longer to produce a certain effect and longer for a single dose to be eliminated from the body.

Some confusion arises over how the various barbiturates are named. In the United States the generic names of the drugs usually end in -al. In Britain, however, the names end in -one. For example, in the United States one barbiturate is called phenobarbital, but in Britain it is called phenobarbitone. The trade names also can vary. For example, hexobarbital is sold in the United States under the name Sombulex; in Switzerland it is called Evipan.

But under all their various names, the barbiturates remain indispensable in the treatment of sleep disorders, epilepsy, and, to a lesser extent now, anxiety. They are also effective as anesthetics for many surgical procedures. Furthermore, for decades barbiturates have been useful in medical and pharmacological research. They still serve as standards by which many new drugs are compared, and their predictable effects make them particularly useful in many research applications. When new sedative-type drugs are developed, for example, they are generally compared to the barbiturates to determine their relative effectiveness.

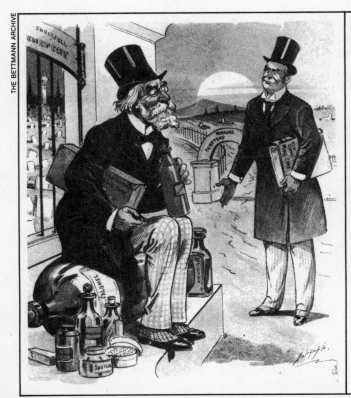

This early cartoon illustrates an ongoing debate in the medical community about the extent to which doctors should rely on the use of drugs in treating patients. Although barbiturates were originally developed to alleviate anxiety and insomnia, it quickly became apparent that there were several serious, even potentially lethal, side effects to these medicines.

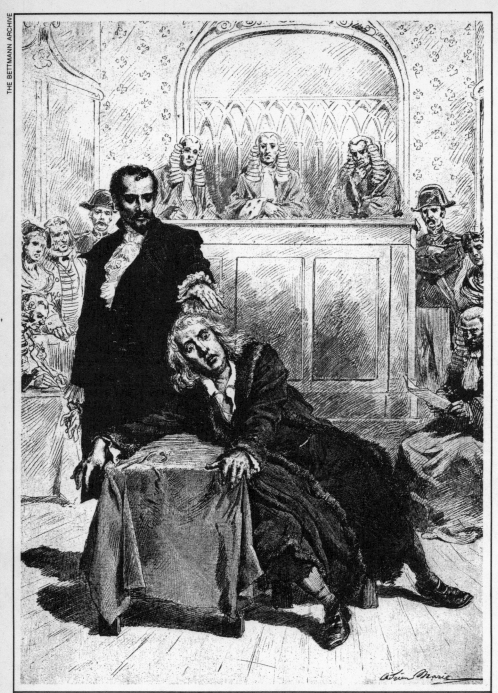

A confession being obtained through hypnosis, in a 19th-century cartoon. Barbiturates are "hypnotic" because they depress the central nervous system in ways that can cause a trance-like state.

CHAPTER 2

HOW DO BARBITURATES WORK?

*T*here have been many studies on the ways in which barbiturates affect the central nervous system. Many such studies have involved applying barbiturates directly to the brain tissue of laboratory animals (usually rats and mice), and measuring the drugs' effects on various brain activities.

The brain is made up of a large number of different types of nerve cells, called neurons. These neurons pass messages to each other by releasing a chemical substance (neurotransmitter) into a space (synaptic cleft) between them (see Figure 1). Some neurotransmitters increase neuron activity; others decrease it. Studies have found, to put a highly complex and technical process very simply, that sedative barbiturates block nerve impulses at these nerve-cell connections. In other words, they act in various ways to decrease neuron activity in the brain.

As we have said, most barbiturates are derived from barbituric acid. There is also a class of barbiturates formed from thiourea, which, unlike barbituric acid, has a sulphur molecule in it. In pharmacological terms, barbiturates formed from thiourea are called thiobarbiturates; barbiturates formed from barbituric acid are called oxybarbiturates. By modifying barbituric acid and thiourea in the laboratory, chemists can create various barbiturates with particular properties and effects. For example, the specific chemical structure of a barbituric acid derivative will determine how quickly the drug will take effect, how long this effect will last, and how much must be taken to induce sleep.

Different barbiturates take effect at different rates and the duration of these effects varies from barbiturate to barbiturate. These differences are determined by two factors:

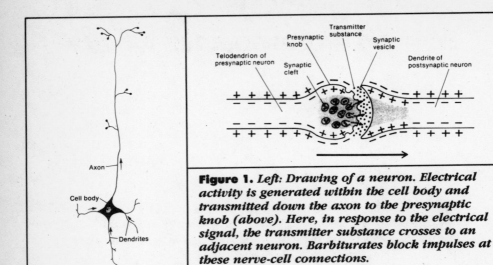

Figure 1. *Left: Drawing of a neuron. Electrical activity is generated within the cell body and transmitted down the axon to the presynaptic knob (above). Here, in response to the electrical signal, the transmitter substance crosses to an adjacent neuron. Barbiturates block impulses at these nerve-cell connections.*

1. how quickly a particular chemical compound reaches the brain; and 2. how quickly the body terminates any particular compound's action. (The action of a barbituric compound is terminated when it reaches the body's fat stores, and/or when it is metabolized by the liver.) The process by which a drug is absorbed and distributed throughout the body and changed (metabolized) by and excreted from the body is called pharmacokinetics. The dynamics of pharmacokinetics are quite complicated, involving such things as the rate at which a drug reaches the part of the body it acts upon, the amounts of it that lodge in nerve, muscle, and fat cells, and the amount of time it lingers in the body before being excreted in the urine. Pharmacokinetics explains many of the differences among barbiturates. For example, methohexital can induce sleep within 1 minute, while phenobarbital takes about 15 minutes to achieve the same result.

Similarly the effects of a barbiturate wear off according to the specific chemical properties of the drug being administered. With ultra-short-acting barbiturates, the first phase of their action ends when the drug moves from the brain to other body tissues. In 15 to 30 minutes, a short-acting drug like thiopental will have been distributed to muscle and skin as well as to the heart, liver, and other similar organs. In an hour it will have been redistributed to the body's fat stores. As muscle and fat absorb the drug, it diffuses out of the brain.

After 30 minutes the brain and the visceral organs may have given up as much as 90% of their initial concentrations.

Drugs that have not yet been changed, or metabolized, by the body remain in the body for hours and may continue to produce what is called a drug hangover. This means it would be dangerous to give more doses of an ultra-short-acting barbiturate to prolong anesthesia. This could lead to overdose.

Except for barbital (Barbital Sodium), barbiturates are mainly metabolized by the liver, and the results of the metabolism are excreted in the urine. Thiobarbiturates, to some extent, are also transformed in other tissues, mainly in the kidneys and brain. Only barbital leaves the body unchanged in urine.

Different barbiturates are metabolized and eliminated from the body at widely different rates. For example, half of a total dose of the long-acting barbiturate phenobarbital will be eliminated in about five days. But half of a total dose of the ultra-short-acting barbiturate hexobarbital is eliminated in five or six hours.

Tolerance and Dependence

Soon after barbital began to be used clinically, the medical community discovered that repeated administration of the drug led to physical dependence. Today we have standardized laboratory procedures to test new drugs, but at that time, in the early 20th century, drugs were "tested" only on patients. As a result, many effects, including dependence potential, were not known prior to actual use.

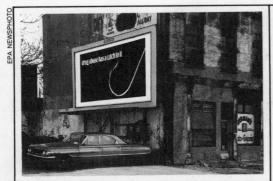

EPA NEWSPHOTO

An anti-drug poster in Philadelphia. One of the "catches" of barbiturate use is tolerance: an individual who regularly takes these drugs for their sedative/ hypnotic effect finds that over time, the original dose loses its effectiveness and ever-increasing doses are required to produce the original effect.

Since drug tolerance—which involves a decreased response to a drug after repeated use—and drug dependence go hand in hand, an individual who regularly takes barbiturates for their sedative-hypnotic effect finds that after a while the original dose is not as effective as it used to be, and that it takes a larger amount of the drug to produce the original effect. The body has thus developed a tolerance to the drug. This is usually accompanied by a growing physiological dependence. As the amounts taken become larger and larger, the likelihood of severe withdrawal symptoms when the individual abruptly stops taking the drug also increases.

That barbiturates could trigger the cycle of tolerance and dependence characteristic of many addictive drugs was observed by researchers working as long ago as the 1930s. One psychiatrist, reporting on the relationship between barbiturates and sleep, observed that "a dose [of Amytal Sodium] which has usually kept a patient soundly asleep for a certain length of time will be insufficient to bring about the same effect later." (This doctor was using barbiturates in a form of psychiatric treatment called sleep therapy. In such therapy, a psychiatric patient was kept sedated for days at a time through the administration of repeated doses of Amytal Sodium. This form of treatment is now completely discredited.) He went on to say that when the sleep therapy was ended

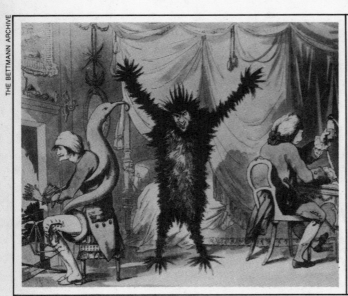

This cartoon of a psychiatric patient suffering from hallucinations somewhat exaggerates the divorce from reality that is a symptom of barbiturate withdrawal. Other manifestations include convulsions, delirium, and extremely high fever.

and administration of the drug was stopped abruptly, it was not unusual to see convulsions in the patients.

The development of tolerance is related to the length of time between administrations of a barbiturate. This is an interval that varies with the duration of action of particular barbiturates. (The shorter the duration of action, the more frequently the drug would have to be administered for tolerance to develop.) Studies with laboratory animals have shown that tolerance can develop in a matter of days when the drug is administered at high doses. When lower doses are given regularly, tolerance will also develop; it just takes longer to reach its peak.

Withdrawal Syndrome

Other studies (using rhesus monkeys) have documented the characteristics and the severity of the barbiturate withdrawal syndrome. A mild withdrawal syndrome includes apprehension, high-excitability, mild tremors, loss of appetite, and piloerection (hair standing on end). An intermediate withdrawal syndrome includes severe tremors, muscle rigidity, impaired motor activity, retching and vomiting, and significant weight loss. A severe withdrawal syndrome includes convulsions, delirium or hallucinations, and hyperthermia, or unusually high fever. The same patterns of reaction to barbiturate withdrawal have been observed in humans.

The severity of the withdrawal syndrome has been shown, like tolerance development, to depend on the frequency of barbiturate administration and the duration of action of the drug. If taken frequently, short- or intermediate-acting barbiturates, like pentobarbital or secobarbital, will be more likely to produce severe physiological dependence than will ultra-short-acting barbiturates, like thiopental. This is because there will still be an appreciable amount of the faster-acting barbiturates in the nervous system at the time of the next dose, even though many of their observable effects may have worn off.

The long-acting barbiturates, like phenobarbital, produce less severe signs when they are withdrawn. Because it takes much longer for them to be eliminated from the body, the body has time to readjust gradually to their absence after the last dose has been taken.

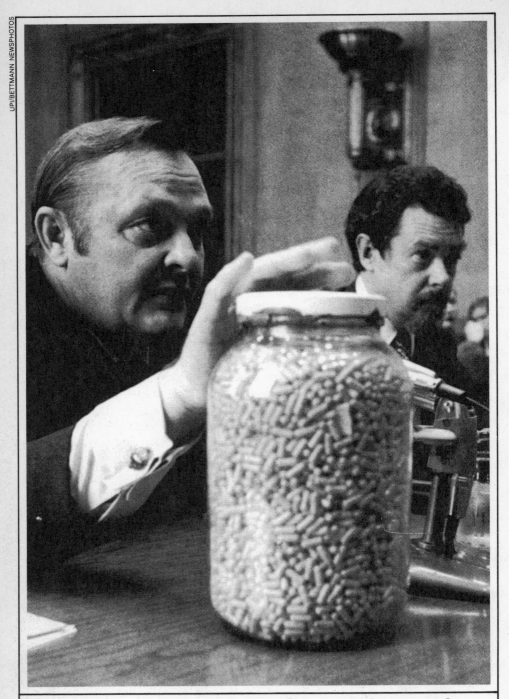

A Los Angeles County district attorney testifies at a 1972 hearing on the problem of barbiturate abuse. In the mid-1970s about 10 thousand patients per year entered treatment centers for abuse of these drugs.

CHAPTER 3

WHAT ARE
THE EFFECTS OF BARBITURATES?

*T*he general effects of barbiturates on mood and behavior were best measured and described more than three decades ago in a study conducted in Lexington, Kentucky by the U.S. Public Health Service. Conducted during the 1950s, this is the only controlled study of barbiturate dependence in humans. It made clear the seriousness of barbiturate abuse at a time when objective clinical data on such effects were not available.

A Controlled Study on Human Subjects

Five men who had abused opiates, as well as either barbiturates or alcohol, volunteered to serve as subjects. They were prisoners serving sentences for narcotics violations in the federal prison in Lexington who had been drug-free for at least three months prior to the experiment.

The experiment was divided into five parts:

1. A two- to three-week preliminary assessment of medical and psychological factors.

2. Regular administration of pentobarbital (2 men), secobarbital (2 men), and amobarbital (1 man), which lasted from three to nearly five months, depending on the subject.

3. Withdrawal, a period during which barbiturates were abruptly and completely discontinued, which lasted from one to two weeks.

4. Recovery, a period that varied from two to four months and during which the men were assessed medically and psychologically. The men lived in dormitories during this period.

5. Reintoxication, a period of only two or three days during which the men were given the same dosages they had received in phase 2.

Many of the effects of the prolonged administration of the barbiturates were the same as those observed after large single doses. These included impairment of mental ability, confusion, regression of personality, emotional instability, rapid and involuntary rolling of the eyeballs, unsteadiness when walking, and slower abdominal reflexes.

But there were some consequences with the prolonged dosages not observed in single doses. One was an apparent accumulation of the drug and the effects of that accumulation. For instance, low doses which previously had little effect caused severe drunkenness after prolonged administration. These cumulative effects were even more pronounced if the subject had not eaten for several hours before taking the drug. Caloric intake fell by about 10% but body weight increased about 3%. The weight gain probably was caused by reduced physical activity since the men slept about two hours more a day than they had previously. Pulse rates quickened about 10 beats a minute.

None of the men showed psychotic behavior, and they had few disorientation problems, although weird dreams were not uncommon. But emotional swings became more pronounced during phase 2, and the men grew progressively irritable, morose, and quarrelsome. Impaired judgment led to falls, carelessness with cigarettes, and a tendency to take more and more drugs. Some of the men developed mild depression and paranoia. Some became sloppy and disorganized in caring for their appearance and health.

One man, designated as S-1, acted as follows:

> Though occasionally euphoric, garrulous, and pleasant, S-1 was usually depressed, complained of various aches and pains and continually sought increases in medication, despite being so intoxicated that he could not walk. He would weep over his wasted life and the state of his family. He became infantile and persuaded his friend, S-2, to carry him to bed, button his clothes, and feed

him. S-1 frequently asked to be released from the experiment but would always change his mind within 30 minutes of missing a dose.

In general, prolonged barbiturate use produces effects similar to those of alcohol and opiates. One difference is that barbiturate users seem to maintain a more stable diet.

As noted earlier, when barbiturate administration is abruptly ended, a distinct withdrawal syndrome emerges. Signs of intoxication disappear, but the user is left physically weak, anxious, and shaky. Loss of appetite, nausea, and vomiting also occur. Pulse and breathing rates quicken. Fever and increased blood pressure, which in turn lead to dizziness and fainting, are also common.

In the Lexington experiments, some of the men suffered serious convulsions and even developed a short-term psychosis similar to the delirium tremens that sometimes affects alcoholics during withdrawals. They experienced anxiety, agitation, insomnia, disorientation, delusions, and hallucinations. Nonetheless, two months after the experiment there was no evidence of permanent damage.

Here is part of the report on how the men reacted:

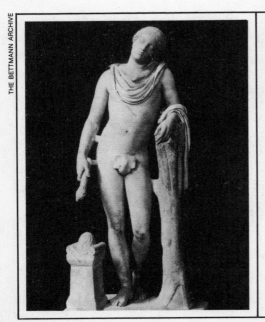

An ancient statue of Hypnos, the Roman god of sleep. Although it was originally hoped that barbiturates would be "miracle drugs" in the treatment of sleep disorders, problems involving their abuse soon proved otherwise.

THE BETTMANN ARCHIVE

During the fourth night of withdrawal, S-1 lay awake giggling in a silly fashion, staring at the walls and talking with nonexistent persons. At this time he was oriented for time, place, and person, and, despite the unmistakable evidence, denied that he was experiencing hallucinations. During the following day he was very apprehensive and occasionally shouted, "Who's that out there?" or, "Did you call me?" He attempted to wash the walls of the rooms, though he had no water and no washcloth. He remained generally well oriented in the major spheres of time ("What is the date?"), place ("Where are you?"), and setting ("Why are you here?"). During the fifth night of withdrawal the psychosis became more severe. He thought that a railroad ran through the ward. He "conversed" with the trainmen about repairs to the locomotive and fantasized making trips to South Carolina with a trainload of goats. On the following day he was once again oriented in time, place, and person but remained apprehensive and frightened and begged for morphine and barbiturates. He admitted that he had been experiencing hallucinations and appeared to realize that they were imaginary and not real. During the sixth night of withdrawal he became disoriented in time and place but not in person. He thought that he was in various places in South Carolina and that he was riding a train; he became agitated because he

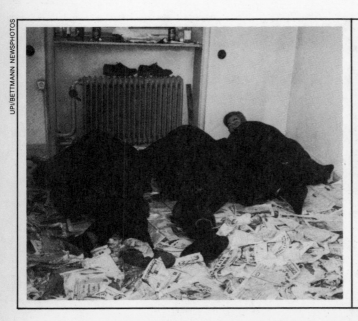

Barbiturate addiction can lead to wild emotional swings, intense irritability, impaired judgment, and the kind of dramatic indifference to personal hygiene characterized by these men in a Stockholm flophouse.

imagined that persons were trying to harm him. He claimed he was blown up three times, was cut by knives, and suffered other forms of violent persecution; several imaginary persons were murdered during the night; he saw tiny men descending in parachutes; an old woman was perched on the ceiling of the room; shimmering rings of light or smoke which floated in the air went in one of his ears, and he pulled them out the other ear. He misidentified persons and objects. During the seventh day he was disoriented in time and place but retained his identity. He had visual and auditory hallucinations constantly, was extremely agitated, and constantly tried to escape from his imaginary persecutors. He stated the belief that one of the physicians and two of the attendants had done various evil things to him, and he threatened them with bodily harm and persecution for their crimes. All these symptoms persisted unabated until the ninth night. At that time, the patient was very excited; he had a temperature of 38.3°C (100.9°F) and a pulse rate of 140. It appeared that he was becoming dangerously exhausted, so withdrawal was terminated.

He was given secobarbital sodium and eventually went to sleep. Hallucinations occurred infrequently during the first day but were gone by the second day. Nevertheless the man still believed that the hallucinations were real and asked that police be called to investigate the murders he had seen. On the third day after being returned to drug dosages he recognized his hallucinations for what they were and was greatly relieved. This time, the dosages of barbiturates were reduced gradually over a period of 34 days. The convulsions and psychosis did not recur.

The man designated S-2 had helped his fellow prisoner, S-1, but had his own problems during the withdrawal phase. He had no convulsions but slept only a little during the third and fourth nights of this stage. At 3 o'clock in the morning on the fifth day he woke up and demanded that a doctor examine him. He said he had "knots" in his head and in his muscles. He claimed that his brain had been jarred loose and had fallen down into his body. He wanted an electroencephalogram taken to find out what had happened.

While the electrodes were being attached, he began to laugh, giggle, and speak to nonexistent people. Later, he said that the "brain wave" machine had been reversed and had put brain waves into his head, instead of taking them out. This situation was "remedied" by taking another electroencephalogram. Throughout the day the patient had various auditory and visual hallucinations. He lay quietly grinning and smiling, staring at the wall and talking to nonexistent persons. When questioned sharply, he appeared startled, stopped watching the wall, answered questions, and, superficially, appeared to be well-oriented. As he answered questions, his attention would wander, he would stare at the wall and stop talking in the middle of a sentence. He imagined seeing women, men, giants, animals and airplanes. He saw himself, or part of himself, on the wall. When asked how he could be in two places at once, he said, "It is funny; I don't see how it is possible, but it is done by a system. They use pictures."

The hallucinations seemed to gain intensity during the day but when night came, the man refused to answer questions. He seemed completely out of touch with reality. He lay on his bed posturing and making faces. He used a pocket comb as a baton as he seemed to be conducting a band. Then he became wildly excited and seemed to be accusing his wife of being unfaithful. At that stage he lost control of his bodily functions and soiled himself.

He spent most of the sixth day of withdrawal watching the walls, laughing, talking to imaginary persons and listening to imaginary music. This behavior continued through the sixth night and through the morning of the seventh day. At noon on the seventh day the patient fell asleep. On awakening, five hours later, he jumped from his bed, eluded the attendants and ran out of the room. He went to the bathroom, washed his face, combed his hair and changed his pajamas. He was hostile and belligerent. He seemed to feel that his hallucinations were associated with the room where he had been kept during withdrawal. He bathed several times, changed pajamas repeatedly and swept the floor. He was allowed to remain in the open ward and after about three hours became calm and again slept. On awakening the next morning, he was not experiencing hallucinations, was quiet, oriented in all spheres, but somewhat hostile and withdrawn.

Later he described some of his hallucinations but claimed he did not remember those involving sex. By the eighth day no sign of psychosis was visible.

The other men involved in the experiments also were visibly affected by the withdrawal from the barbiturates but not quite so dramatically.

During the decades that have passed since the Lexington experiments many other studies have been conducted on the effects of barbiturates. They have generally supported the validity of the observations made in Lexington. Such studies could not easily be repeated now. At that time they were considered models of safe and ethical research. Now, however, greater concern for human rights would almost certainly forbid the use of prisoners, even if they "volunteered" for such studies. Fortunately, the Lexington experiments were conclusive enough so that they do not need to be repeated.

The Mood-Altering Properties of Barbiturates

All tests on the effects of barbiturates point to the conclusion that chronic barbiturate intoxication is dangerous and undesirable. People so affected are confused, unable to think clearly, and have poor judgment and impaired emotional control. Personality defects are accentuated and minor slights and fancied insults engender hostility and rage. They often regress and behave like small children. At times they become depressed to the point of suicide. They frequently fall and injure themselves. They pass out while smoking. They are unable to work and are menaces when driving automobiles. They are prone to taking ever larger doses of barbiturates, leading to overdoses and even to death. Sometimes these deaths are in effect suicides.

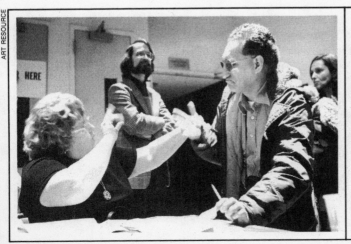

One of the classic side effects of barbiturate addiction involves a serious loss of emotional control. Addicts are often quarrelsome and belligerent, overreacting to imagined insults.

ART RESOURCE

Barbiturates clearly produce diverse changes in mood, emotions, and behavior. The changes are not random. They are closely related to the dosage, to the past drug experience of the user, and to the circumstances in which the drug is used.

For instance, when a person receives the ultra-short-acting barbiturate methohexital (Brevital) to induce loss of consciousness in a dentist's office, recovery may be unpleasant because the patient often has great difficulty recovering self-control. In less stressful surroundings, however, the experience may even seem pleasant. Why do the effects of the barbiturates vary so?

Dosage is perhaps the most critical factor.

Since barbiturates are general depressants of the central nervous system, in high doses they produce sedation and depress body and behavior functions. The body tends to resist changes in some of these functions. This means that the doses have to be high to fight that resistance. For example, if a person is paid for doing a particular job and will lose pay if the job is not done, tolerance will be more likely to develop to the work-disrupting effects of barbiturates.

Other behavior patterns, however, are more easily affected. Thus, someone who is shy and has difficulty in reacting socially will often become more talkative and relaxed after taking a depressant such as a barbiturate or alcohol. Sometimes, however, this can have unfortunate results. For example, a person under the influence of a barbiturate may try

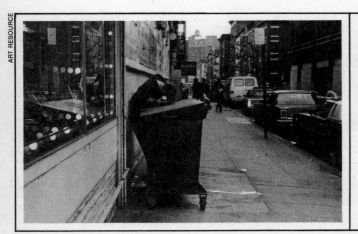

Chronic barbiturate intoxication is dangerous and destructive. People so affected are confused, unable to think clearly, and, at times, depressed to the point of suicide.

to do something dangerous which he or she would not otherwise attempt.

Previous experience can also determine the effects of barbiturate use. For a person not experienced with drugs, the diminished control over mood and behavior that is produced by a sedative can be most unpleasant. However, familiarity with the effects of drugs in certain social situations can breed enjoyment of those effects. If someone deliberately uses drugs to avoid unpleasantness, similar agreeable feelings can be attained.

Their tendency to lower inhibitions led to barbiturates being used as "truth serums," the idea being that under the influence of barbiturates people would readily reveal carefully guarded secrets. Although the serums did indeed have that effect in some cases, in others they were just as likely to inspire pure fabrications and fantasies.

To examine the effects of barbiturates on mood, a study was conducted by the Addiction Research Center in Baltimore. Twelve men with histories of alcohol and sedative abuse volunteered to take part. During the eight-week study the subjects lived at the research center. On test days they were given either a placebo, one of several dosages of pentobarbital (the most commonly studied "standard" barbiturate), or one of several dosages of Valium, a non-barbiturate, for comparison. Neither the staff who administered the drug and measured its effects nor the patients were told the nature of the dose. The study yielded a great deal of valuable information about physical and behavorial responses to the varying dosages.

Both pentobarbital and Valium produced similar general reactions; both had sedative and euphoric effects and both intensified such negative feelings as tiredness and emotional instability. Observers reported that the patients seemed to "like" the way both drugs made them feel despite undesirable side effects such as slurred speech and lack of coordination.

The main difference between the two drugs involved the dosages required to produce the particular effects. Valium was effective at lower doses. Another difference between the two drugs is more subtle; Valium was a little slower to act but its effects lasted longer than pentobarbital's effects.

The study once again showed that the effects of barbiturates are not random. They are related to the amount taken and to the amount of time between dosages. In the same patients, Valium and the barbiturates could each act as depressants or stimulants. But Valium use was found to be less likely to lead to overdoses. Moreover, Valium's unique properties make it particularly valuable in clinical medicine.

Barbiturates and Driving Don't Mix

Although barbiturates have many medical benefits, they also have their drawbacks. Nowhere is this more apparent than when they are used in conjunction with driving an automobile. The effects of sedatives on a driver's judgment can be devastating. A driver depends on his senses to drive safely. His or her sense of sight is especially important. Under the influence of barbiturates, however, a driver is often unable to judge distance and speed and to adapt to changing light conditions. An accident can easily result. Even the sense of touch can be adversely affected. A driver under the influence of barbiturates can be too slow to apply the brakes or too quick to put his or her foot on the accelerator. Sedatives can also slow a driver's responses even if a sensory cue has been properly detected. Subtle changes in muscle coordination may be particularly devastating if driving conditions are hazardous or if traffic is heavy. Several scientific studies have proven that barbiturates do indeed impair performance and produce errors that could lead to fatal accidents.

Similar findings were obtained in a study using flight simulators. Use of secobarbital impaired skills critical to the safe operation of an airplane. In these tests, however, testing did not begin until 10 hours after the drug had been given and then continued over 12 more hours. The most important test result may have been that poor performances continued throughout the testing. In other words, nearly 24 hours after the drug had been administered it was still impairing pilot performance. This was much longer that the typically observed peak effects of what is considered to be a short-acting barbiturate.

In a recent automobile driving simulator test, a screen was placed in front of the test car. A programmed sequence simulated driving under country and city conditions. Changing traffic lights, changes in course, and an emergency situation in which another car drove into the path of the test car were simulated.

In this study two barbiturates were given in the way that they might be administered for a routine surgical procedure such as a tooth extraction. A pre-anesthetic, atropine sulfate, was given followed by an injection of either thiopental or methohexital. The tests were conducted 2, 4, 6, and 8 hours after the drugs were injected.

Before each stage of the tests, the drivers were questioned about how they felt in general and how they felt about their driving ability. At the 2-hour stage, most drivers felt impaired. At the 4-hour stage, only about half felt impaired. By 6 or 8 hours most drivers thought their skills were back to normal.

The actual tests showed that performance on such things as brake reaction time did improve with time but other errors continued well past the 8-hour stage. As in the flight simulator study, the poor performance level persisted well beyond the time typically ascribed to these drugs, which in this case were ultra-short-acting barbiturates.

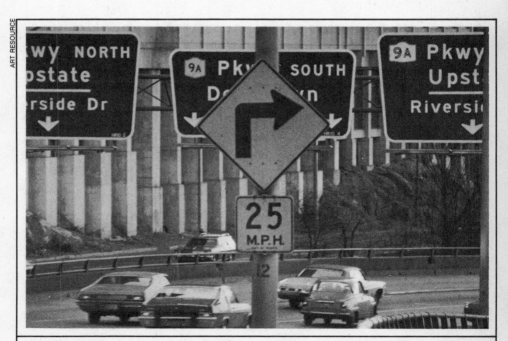

Maximum alertness and quick reflexes are required for the safe handling of a motor vehicle. Numerous scientific studies have proven that barbiturates dangerously impair driving ability.

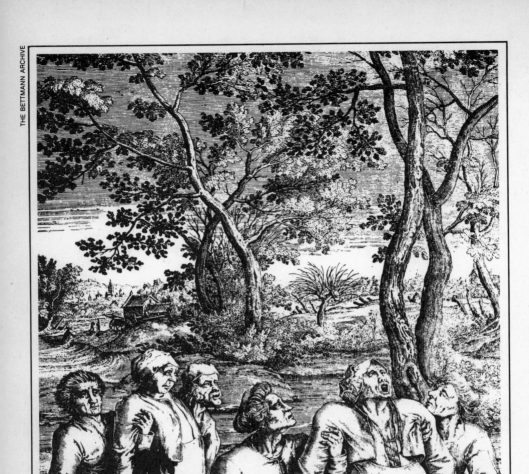

F.B. inv.   *H. sculp*

Two victims of epilepsy before the advent of modern medical treatments. The discovery of the barbiturate phenobarbital was a great breakthrough in the treatment of epilepsy and other convulsive disorders.

CHAPTER 4

WHAT ARE THE MEDICAL USES OF BARBITURATES?

Barbiturates are sold in a wide variety of preparations. Alone or in mixtures, they can be bought as powders, elixirs, syrups, drops, capsules, tablets, or suppositories. Many of these barbiturates, for example, amobarbital (Amytal) and pentobarbital sodium (Nembutal Sodium), are also available in injectable forms. The ultra-short-acting barbiturates are marketed only in the injectable form.

Barbiturates are prescribed for almost any condition in which it is necessary to depress the central nervous system. The effects of barbiturates range from anticonvulsant-sedative action at lower doses, to hypnosis, anesthesia, poisoning, and even death, as the dose is increased. Theoretically, any of these effects can be produced by any barbiturate, but practically speaking, each barbiturate is chemically distinct from the others. Because of their chemical differences, different amounts of each barbiturate are needed to produce each effect. As a result, the barbiturates have specialized uses. The biggest difference in clinical use is between the ultra-short-acting barbiturates and all of the others. Because ultra-short-acting barbiturates have such quick and controllable effects, they are used almost exclusively in an intravenous form to produce anesthesia during surgery. If the patient begins to awaken during surgery, the anesthesiologist can use an ultra-short-acting barbiturate to sedate him to a satisfactory level within a few seconds. The ultra-short-acting barbiturates are so useful as analgesics (painkillers) that they are also known as the "anesthetic" barbiturates.

Barbiturates as Tranquilizers and Sleeping Pills

The short-acting and intermediate-acting barbiturates are used most often as sedatives or tranquilizers and for their hypnotic or sleep-inducing effects. They are especially useful as hypnotics since, when taken orally (usually in pill or capsule form), they act within a few minutes. If the dose is right they produce a moderate-to-deep sleep that lasts all night. Occasional use of barbiturates to induce sleep is invaluable for patients who are unable to sleep because of acute pain or trauma (a condition of severe shock following a physical or emotional blow). Repeated use of barbiturates as sedatives or sleeping pills, however, may lead to dependence or to deep disturbances in sleeping patterns.

The long-acting barbiturates are used more often as sedatives than as hypnotics. They require a longer time to take effect and a longer time to wear off. This makes them less

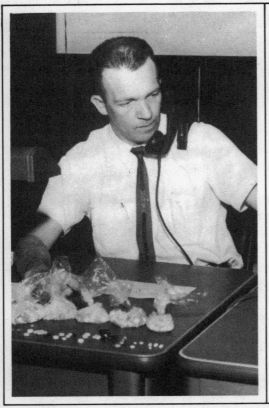

UPI/BETTMANN NEWSPHOTOS

A police officer displays a cache of barbiturates that were seized before they could be distributed illegally. Barbiturates are manufactured as capsules, powders, elixirs, syrups, drops, tablets, and suppositories.

disruptive to the patient's everyday life. If the dose of a long-acting barbiturate is correct, patients can often function very well at many ordinary tasks, as long as they do not require peak functioning and coordination.

Barbiturates as Anticonvulsants

The most useful application of the long-acting barbiturates is in the treatment of certain forms of epilepsy. Phenobarbital, for example, is frequently employed for this purpose. For many patients who have occasional grand mal epileptic seizures (uncontrolled convulsions or fits), it is possible to find a dose of phenobarbital that produces little sedation and causes minor loss of coordination, but is nevertheless strong enough to prevent the seizures.

Phenobarbital is the oldest anticonvulsant drug still in use. Shortly after its first clinical use in 1912, it proved to be more effective in treating some kinds of seizures than the bromide drugs previously used. There are a number of dif-

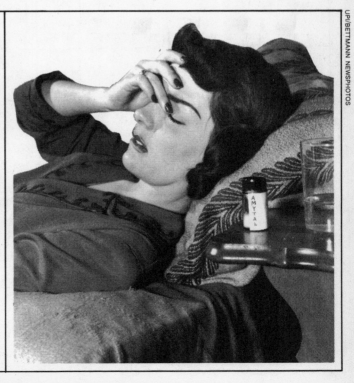

A woman experiencing the onset of barbiturate poisoning. When tolerance to the sedative effects of barbiturates develops, higher dosages of the drug are needed in order to achieve the original effects. This kind of situation can lead to barbiturate overdose and acute, sometimes fatal, results.

UPI/BETTMANN NEWSPHOTOS

Table 2

Some of the Most Common Barbiturates		
GENERIC NAME	TRADE NAME	RECOMMENDED USES
Long-Acting Barbiturates		
barbital	Veronal or Neuronidia	sedative
mephobarbital	Mebaral	anticonvulsant; sedative
metharbital	Gemonil	anticonvulsant
phenobarbital	Solfoton	sedative; anticonvulsant
Short- and Intermediate-Acting Barbiturates		
amobarbital	Amytal	sedative; preanesthetic
amobarbital sodium	Amytal Sodium	sedative; anticonvulsant*; narco-therapy; narco-analysis; diagnostic aid in schizophrenia
butabarbital	Butisol	sedative; insomnia
aprobarbital	Alurate	insomnia
pentobarbital sodium	Nembutal Sodium	sedative; insomnia; preanesthetic; anticonvulsant*
secobarbital	Seconal	insomnia; hypnosis
talbutal	Lotusate	sedative; hypnosis
amobarbital sodium and secobarbital sodium in equal parts	Tuinal	insomnia
Ultra-Short-Acting Barbiturates		
hexobarbital	Sombulex	intravenous anesthetic
methohexital	Brevital	intravenous anesthetic; inducing hypnosis
thiamylal	Surital	intravenous anesthetic; inducing hypnosis
thiopental	Pentothal	intravenous anesthetic; anticonvulsant*; narco-analysis

*emergency treatment of seizures

ferent types of epileptic seizures, and some drugs control one kind better than others. But since a patient may suffer from two or more kinds of seizures, multiple drugs frequently are given. Phenobarbital is especially useful in treating grand mal seizures and cortical focal seizures. It calms the convulsion at dosages that produce minimal sedation. This is not true of most other barbiturates, however. They would have to be given at such high doses that the patient would be deeply sedated.

Phenobarbital is also the least toxic of the barbiturates. In addition, it is probably the cheapest treatment for prolonged treatment of seizures. While other alternative medicines, many of them structurally related to phenobarbital, have recently been developed, phenobarbital remains widely used.

The way in which anti-epileptic drugs work is still not completely understood. It is thought that most of them prevent normal nerve cells from being excited by abnormal neurons that cause seizures. The barbiturates may very well sedate these neurons, thus making them less prone to produce or prolong seizures.

Two other long-acting barbiturates also have been used for treating seizures. One is mephobarbital (Mebaral), which in the body is converted to phenobarbital. Because the ab-

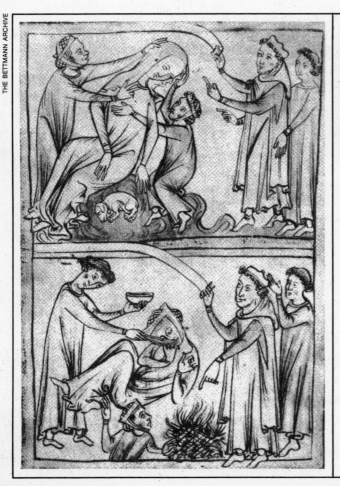

*A **medieval drawing** depicts **Saint Valentine** **curing epileptics**. It is believed that barbiturates are effective in controlling diseases such as epilepsy because they sedate abnormal neurons that cause seizures.*

sorption of mephobarbital is less complete than that of pheno-barbital, it is therefore less potent. Metharbital (Gemonil) also changes once in the body—to barbital. It is especially effective for treating a particular spasmodic ailment found in children.

Complications in the Treatment of Insomnia and Anxiety

For many years, barbiturates were commonly used to treat insomnia: they do effectively induce a sound sleep that can be maintained for up to seven hours. Unfortunately, it soon became apparent that the routine use of barbiturates to induce sleep could cause some rather severe problems. First, patients found it necessary to take larger and larger doses of the drugs to achieve the same effects. The former dosage lost its power as the patient developed a tolerance to the drug. Because of this, it is now recommended that the use of secobarbital (Seconal) and pentobarbital sodium (Nembutal Sodium) be discontinued after two weeks of nightly use. Otherwise, the patient may independently increase his prescribed dose in the ongoing battle to get a good night's sleep. This can lead to a strong and very dangerous dependence on the drug.

Another potentially severe problem that can result from the regular use of barbiturates is that tolerance to the drug may develop to the point at which the dosage, to be effective, reaches an extremely dangerous level. While the body is developing tolerance to certain of the effects, it is *not* developing tolerance to the lethal effect of the drugs. In other words, the clinically effective dose eventually becomes very close to the lethal dose. For this reason, barbiturate overdose often results in an acute, sometimes fatal, medical emergency.

For these reasons a newer class of drugs, the benzodiazepines, of which Valium and Librium are the prototypes, has been developed. These drugs can also produce dependence but are far less lethal than the barbiturates unless used in combination with other sedatives. Also, the withdrawal process is not as likely to be as life-threatening as it is with barbiturates. But even with these newer drugs, doctors more and more are seeking to discourage anything other than temporary use.

Barbiturates used as hypnotics can also be used for daytime sedation when the dosage is cut to one-third or one-quarter of the nighttime dose. Barbiturates, particularly phenobarbital, were once used almost exclusively in such treatment. But now drugs such as Valium and Librium have largely supplanted them.

Phenobarbital and amobarbital have been used to treat anxiety. But since anxiety may go hand-in-hand with depression, the possibility of suicide arises. For this reason, the high toxicity of the barbiturates again makes them less preferred than the benzodiazepines.

Multi-Drug Therapies

Sometimes, to avoid dependence, doctors will switch patients from barbiturates to other drugs. In many instances, such changes are indeed beneficial, especially for patients suffering from anxiety. But the changes are not without potential danger. For instance, a study at The Johns Hopkins University School of Medicine discovered that mood and social behavior may deteriorate during periods of prolonged use of drugs from the family to which Valium and Librium belong.

Phenobarbital and butalbital are sometimes prescribed in combination with other drugs for treatment of stress, tension, or muscle contraction headaches. The other components typically are acetaminophen or aspirin, and sometimes caffeine as well. Some preparations with butabarbital also include codeine or hydrocodone to provide additional pain-killing effects.

Phenobarbital is included in a number of preparations used to treat bowel ailments and duodenal (intestinal) ulcer problems. In this case, the other components are belladonna alkaloids, which function as antispasmodics. The phenobarbital is included to act as a mild sedative.

In some preparations for treating bronchial asthma, bronchitis, bronchospasm, and emphysema, butabarbital or phenobarbital are included. They may be combined in this case with an expectorant or drugs such as theophylline or ephedrine that dilate the bronchia. In addition to acting as sedatives the barbiturates also act to decrease the effects of the ephedrine, which sometimes may produce jitteriness in a patient.

Butabarbital is also used in a preparation for treating urinary tract inflammation. Pentobarbital's sedative effects are sometimes used in preparations to combat nausea. Phenobarbital is included in a preparation with enzymes to aid digestion. It is also used to decrease the frequency and severity of attacks of angina pectoris (severe pain and constriction about the heart) when anxiety or emotional disturbances are present. Barbiturates have also long been used for treating seizures.

Barbiturates as Anesthetics

Barbital, the first barbiturate, was originally used as an intravenous anesthetic. It was soon replaced, however, by thiopental (Pentothal), which acted more quickly than the longer-acting barbital. But, although the short- and ultra-short-acting barbiturates put their patients to sleep faster, and their effects also wear off more rapidly, they are also actually eliminated more slowly from the body. For this reason they tend to produce an unpleasant drug hangover following anesthesia. In addition, they slow respiration (a dangerous characteristic of all barbiturates). It is true that some other anesthetics such as nitrous oxide have the same effect, but they can be administered with more careful adjustments.

Generally, barbiturates are now used in conjunction with inhalant anesthetics, although they may also be used alone for very short procedures such as tooth extractions, because the short-acting barbiturates, like Brevital, achieve both deep sleep and a return to consciousness in a short period of time. Introduced in 1957, methohexital (Brevital) is about three times as potent for producing anesthesia as thiopental and is now popular for dental and other minor surgery. Both these agents produce a state of anesthesia within minutes after injection. Thiopental and methohexital are still the standards by which all intravenous anesthetics are judged.

Psychiatric Uses of Barbiturates

In the 1930s barbiturates were used in the United States and Europe to induce sleep during sleep therapy sessions. Such procedures had first been described as early as the mid-1800s. There were different theories as to why the therapy would work and many opinions about how successful it was. Many doctors believed that it allowed a disturbed patient to retreat into a "protected state." Others thought that the drug produced beneficial changes in the body's metabolism. Still others felt that the treatment produced a "mellowing of the psyche," making a patient more receptive to psychiatric treatment.

Alcohol, opium, ether, and chloroform, as well as various mixtures of each, have all been used to induce sleep, but after the introduction of barbiturates they were gradually replaced. Amobarbital sodium (Amytal Sodium), synthesized around 1927, was particularly used for therapy. In one psychiatric clinic, patients diagnosed as having reactive depression (a psychosis resulting from abnormal grief and sadness, or a situation causing such emotions), manic depression, and schizophrenia were given doses of Amytal Sodium sufficient to keep them asleep for days at a time. The shortest period of sleep was three days. The longest was 27 days and the average about 11 days. Dosages had to be increased to keep

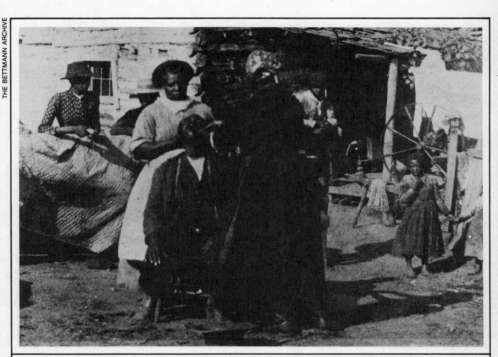

A late 19th-century photograph of a woman extracting her husband's tooth. Short-acting barbiturates are now used in dental surgery because they produce deep sleep and then a rapid return to consciousness.

the patients asleep since they developed a tolerance for the drug. Predictable withdrawal symptoms accompanied the end of therapy.

The goal of this therapy was to make psychiatric patients more communicative and receptive to psychotherapy during the periods in which they slumbered in a sort of twilight zone between consciousness and sleep. Hopes for success were raised when it was noted that some patients did become much more communicative when given Amytal Sodium. Eventually, however, this method of treatment proved disappointing and it has been largely abandoned.

But Amytal Sodium still has a place in American psychiatry, especially as a treatment for panic in such cases as

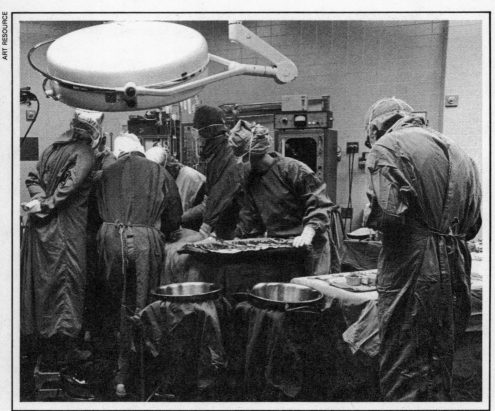

Barbiturates play a significant role as anesthetics in both minor and major surgery. The type of barbiturate used in a surgical procedure depends on how long the patient must remain unconscious.

rape or a traumatic accident. It is also used to break down inhibitions in patients who have trouble talking to a therapist. Some therapists believe that use of Amytal Sodium in an interview facilitates diagnosis when they are dealing with patients who are exhibiting symptoms of both depression and schizophrenia. Even this use of Amytal Sodium, however, is somewhat problematic, because a carefully controlled study comparing the use of Amytal Sodium and a placebo did not support the usefulness of the drug. Patients who had received Amytal Sodium and patients who only thought they had received it but had actually received a salt solution both revealed new information about their lives.

The one type of psychiatric problem for which Amytal Sodium does appear to be unquestionably useful is in the diagnosis of catatonic schizophrenia, a condition in which patients remain mute and stay in fixed positions for a long time. It has been found that such persons respond dramatically to administration of Amytal Sodium. They soon move about, speak, and show interest in their surroundings. The authors of one study of this treatment described the case of a 25-year-old woman:

> On admission, she lay motionless in bed, kept her eyes closed, and would not speak. She required intravenous fluids, an indwelling Foley catheter, and positioning in bed. .... Despite attempts to converse with the patient, these catatonic behaviors persisted for several days. On the sixth hospital day, a total of 350 mg of amobarbital sodium was given intravenously. The patient gradually became more animated as the drug was being administered and began to answer numerous questions in detail. She stated her reluctance to sign the voluntary admission [to the hospital] form and gave a number of reasons why she would not do so. She got up, brushed her teeth, and read a newspaper. As the effect of the barbiturate diminished over the next several hours, she relapsed into the same catatonic state she had been in prior to the injection of amobarbital sodium.

It should be pointed out, however, that although the administration of amobarbital sodium may help a doctor communicate with catatonic schizophrenics, it does not cure them. Such patients revert to mutism (refusal to speak) when the drug wears off.

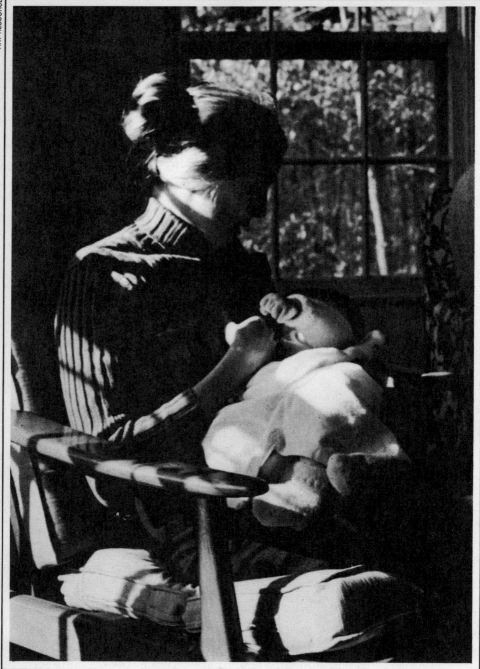

Although barbiturate use during pregnancy has not been specifically linked to birth defects, it is known that short- and ultra-short-acting barbiturates cross the placenta and enter the fetus's bloodstream.

CHAPTER 5

THE RISKS OF BARBITURATE THERAPY

Barbiturates have a number of often predictable side effects that sometimes limit their medical use. For example, when given intravenously as anesthetics, barbiturates often produce a state of excitation before deep anesthesia has been attained. This is characterized by muscle movements and tremors. Mild respiratory upsets such as coughing or hiccupping can also occur during this induction phase.

A few people have also experienced a kind of allergic reaction to barbiturates. Usually they are persons who are sensitive to other drugs or who have a history of asthma, hay fever, or eczema. Given the frequency with which thiopental and methohexital are used, however, the number of such reported cases is minuscule.

In some cases, excitement rather than sedation may occur after the administration of barbiturates. In these cases the patient may even appear drunk. This occurs most often with phenobarbital and similarly structured barbiturates.

At low doses, barbiturates may actually increase some people's susceptibility to pain. And, when given to someone in pain, a barbiturate may cause restlessness, excitement, and even delirium. In some rare cases barbiturates have been known to cause muscular, neuralgic, or arthritic pain. This was most frequently located around the neck, shoulder, and upper arms. The symptoms persisted even after the drug was discontinued.

"Hangover" from relatively small doses of barbiturate has also been noted, particularly from the long-acting barbiturates. Symptoms include tiredness, vertigo, nausea, vomiting, diarrhea, and emotional upsets.

Among those who inject barbiturates severe tissue damage, or necrosis, is a common complication. This happens when the drug is accidentally injected into an artery, rather than a vein.

People with kidney or liver ailments may be especially sensitive to the effects of barbiturates since their bodies may not be able to metabolize and eliminate the drug. For example, a person with hepatitis who takes a barbiturate sleeping pill may stay asleep for an alarmingly long time.

Barbiturate Overdose and Poisoning

Basically, barbiturate overdose results in a state of anesthesia accompanied by general depression of the central nervous system. Typically, breathing is slowed, and that causes a lack of oxygen in the blood. The temperature-regulating center

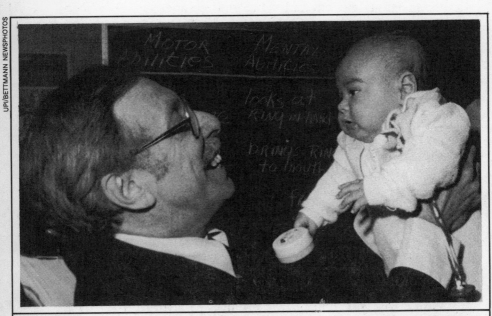

UPI/BETTMANN NEWSPHOTOS

Representative Lester Wolff holds the son of a patient at a New York City narcotics treatment facility. Even when barbiturates are taken under a doctor's supervision, dangerous complications can set in.

in the brain may be affected, causing the body to overcool. Similarly, the heartbeat may slow and blood pressure fall. Finally, shock may set in, either as a direct result of the high dose of barbiturate or because of the other factors. If such a condition occurs outside a hospital, the victim is more likely to die.

Barbiturate poisoning is classified in three categories: mild, moderate, and severe. In mild cases the patient appears to be lightly anesthetized. Muscle reflexes and eye reflexes are present and usually still active. The patient responds to painful stimulation—rubbing the patient's breastbone with the knuckles is a standard test for this. Breathing and blood pressure are normal. In most cases recovery is usually achieved without much trouble.

In moderate poisoning, muscle reflexes may still be present, but generally some eye reflexes will have been lost. The most obvious symptom is a patient's minimal response to painful stimulation. Breathing may be slow but still adequate. Blood pressure remains normal.

In cases of severe poisoning, the patient falls into a deep coma. Muscle and eye reflexes gradually disappear, and there

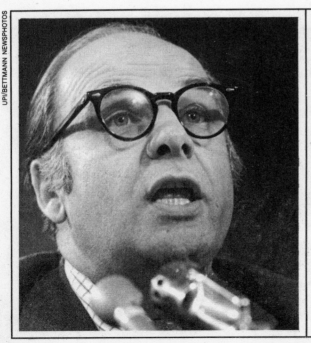

UPI/BETTMANN NEWSPHOTOS

In 1973, Senator Gaylord Nelson urged Congress to restrict the promotion of prescription drugs, an activity on which he claimed the pharmaceutical companies spent a fortune every year. A mixture of barbiturates and other prescription drugs can lead, among other things, to an undesirable level of sedation and to complications in the treatment of overdose.

is no response to painful stimulation. Initially, the face is often reddened. Soon it becomes ashen and finally bluish. Breathing becomes shallow, often slow at first but then rapid. The pulse rate tends to increase and, as the circulation begins to fail, becomes more rapid but of lower volume (less blood flows through the veins). Finally, the pulse can barely be felt. Usually the pupils are constricted but, in contrast to morphine poisoning, they still show some reaction to light; occasionally they are extremely dilated. In serious poisoning, reflexes of the throat and neck muscles are lost. This can lead to the accumulation of mucus in the bronchial tree and eventual respiratory failure. As a result of damage to small blood vessels caused by the reduced blood flow—and perhaps also by toxic action—blisters of the skin and bedsores may develop. The buttocks can be particularly affected in cases where the victim has lain for a long time in the same position. In some rare cases, even in young people, extensive muscle damage to large areas and even entire extremities may occur. This is caused by the immobility of the body, reduced blood circulation, and the pronounced cooling of the body. Unconsciousness from an overdose of phenobarbital may last as long as a week.

Pregnant women run some risk in taking barbiturates. Within a few minutes after the injection of a short- or ultra-short-acting barbiturate, the concentration of barbiturate in the fetus's blood is almost the same as that of the mother's. Because barbiturates are distributed to all body tissues, small amounts may appear in the mother's milk after injection of large barbiturate doses.

Problems can also arise when barbiturates are given in combination with other drugs. For example, when barbiturates are given with another sedative the effect may well be doubled. Combined use of drugs can also complicate the treatment of overdose and dependence. Similarly, the use of barbiturates in combination with another drug may mask the effects of the second drug, further complicating treatment.

Dangers for the Elderly

Barbiturate use among elderly patients potentially presents its own complex of consequences. Although the elderly tend to have problems unique to their stage of life—for example, having to move from their homes into retirement facilities, financial problems, the loss of a spouse—studies have indicated that physicians sometimes fail to take the age of their patients into account when it comes to prescribing drugs. Thus, many elderly persons are given barbiturates when their special problems might better be treated by counseling.

Another problem that is particularly serious for the elderly involves the dangers of falling. It has been established that prescription medications are partly responsible for many of the falls. This is not to say that elderly persons should be denied barbiturates, but rather that their special needs and risks be carefully considered.

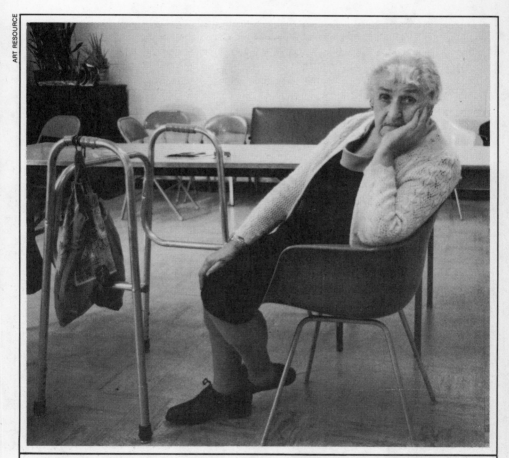

Studies show that physicians often fail to take the age of their patients into account when they prescribe medications. The elderly are particularly vulnerable to the disorienting effects of barbiturates.

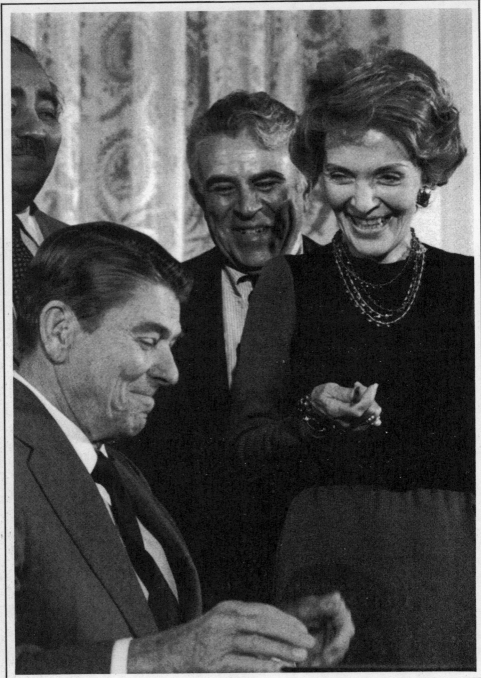

President Ronald Reagan signs a proclamation creating a Drug Abuse Education Week as First Lady Nancy Reagan looks on. Mrs. Reagan has headed a campaign to combat drug abuse among the nation's young people.

CHAPTER 6

HOW ARE BARBITURATES ABUSED?

Since 1973 governmental regulations have increasingly controlled the extent to which barbiturates are prescribed and administered. In that year the Drug Enforcement Administration (DEA) altered the rules by which physicians could dispense pentobarbital, secobarbital sodium, and amobarbital sodium.

The DEA did this by reclassifying the drugs according to the Schedules they use as guidelines for the regulation of drug use. They moved certain barbiturates from Schedule III to Schedule II. The lower the schedule number, the more tightly a drug is controlled. For instance, heroin, LSD, marijuana, and methaqualone are in Schedule I. This means that they are not to be used for general medical purposes in the United States, although they may be used for experiments. Cocaine, morphine, and amphetamines are in Schedule II. This means that these drugs have a high potential for abuse but may be prescribed, subject to special regulations. Schedule III drugs have a lower potential for abuse and may be prescribed at a doctor's discretion. Non-narcotic painkillers and drugs such as Valium are in Schedule IV. Their use is as prescribed by a doctor.

Since the three barbiturates have been placed in Schedule II, prescriptions for them cannot be telephoned to a druggist except in an emergency. In that case a written prescription must be provided to the pharmacist within 72 hours. Refills are not permitted. Other barbiturates are placed in either Schedule III or IV. Though they are dispensed somewhat more freely, a new prescription is still required for each new drug purchase.

How Widespread Is Abuse?

It is often hard to tell how many people in any given population group are actually abusing drugs. Estimates vary but every year the National Institute on Drug Abuse sponsors a national survey on drug use by high school seniors. Participating students from across the country provide a valid picture of current drug use.

According to recent surveys, approximately 15% of high school seniors have tried sedatives at some time in their lives, while about 4% to 5% used them within the previous year. An encouraging trend, however, is that the use of barbiturates and other sedatives has dropped sharply in recent years.

Abuse of barbiturates is not a new phenomenon. Shortly after barbital was introduced in Germany in 1903, case reports of prolonged intoxication and deliberate overdose appeared. By the 1940s abuse of the drugs had become so widespread that magazines such as *Hygeia* and *Collier's* launched a campaign against nonmedical use of barbiturates, or "thrill pills" as they were called. By the 1950s the illicit use of barbiturates was epidemic and was becoming an accepted way to get "high." In the 1960s, use on America's campuses was common. Moreover, abuse of the drugs had spread to adolescents and even younger children, who probably often obtained their supplies from family medicine cabinets. Just how serious the barbiturate problem had become is shown from the fact that in 1964, of 50,400 poison treatment cases in England and Wales, 16,300 involved people who had taken barbiturates.

Many young people used barbiturates in combination with other drugs. In some instances they were taken before the injection of a narcotic on the false assumption that this would heighten or enhance its effect. Or they were taken in combination with amphetamines in an attempt to lessen the agitation that amphetamines produce. There was little scientific basis, however, for such expectations. Rather, barbiturates used in combination with other drugs resulted in many deaths from overdoses. Furthermore, the intravenous use of barbiturates common in the drug subcultures of the 1960s often led to abscesses, destruction of tissue around the injection site, and even death, since the margin between the desired effect and overdose is very narrow.

The 1970s and 1980s have witnessed a decline in barbiturate abuse. By 1975 the Domestic Council Drug Abuse Task Force reported that while 300,000 regular users of barbiturates were "in trouble," illicit use of the drugs by young people had levelled off in the previous three years. In 1984 a report on adolescent drug use in the *American Journal of Public Health* referred to barbiturates as "has-been" drugs.

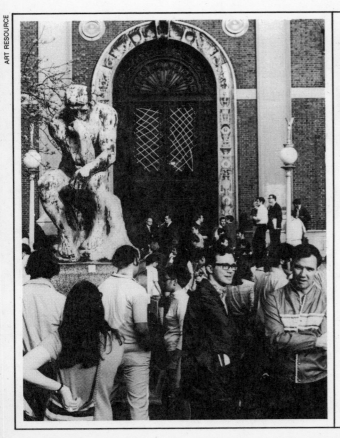

A late 1960s anti-war demonstration at New York City's Columbia University. Barbiturate abuse, which reached epidemic proportions during the 1950s, was still common on college campuses a decade later.

ART RESOURCE

Intentional Overdosing

But for those who still do abuse barbiturates, the dangers cannot be overstated. The most severe risks involve the possibility of overdosing, either accidentally or intentionally. Profiles of people who overdose with drugs generally show that they have poor relationships with the principal figures in their lives. For married people, this typically means that the victims are involved in "a bad marriage." In addition, they frequently are separated or divorced from their spouses. One writer characterized the situation in this way:

> More than any other factor these bad personal relationships . . . provided the setting for the self-poisoning act. Yet in many cases they but set the seal on a life pattern characterized by adverse circumstances—a bad work record, chronic debt, and constant changes of home. . . .

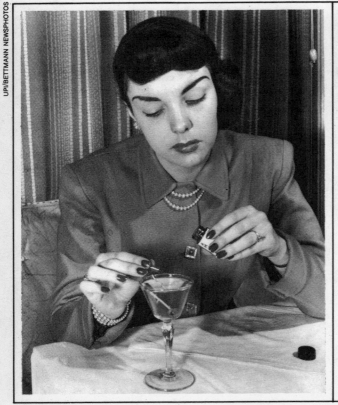

This woman is mixing barbiturates with alcohol. This is an extremely dangerous combination, since both subtances act as central nervous system depressants.

UPI/BETTMANN NEWSPHOTOS

Moreover, these life stories seemed to repeat similar stories in the parents' lives and there had been a great amount of parental absence during the childhood of the patients.

Although some experts feel that anyone who deliberately overdoses must be mentally disturbed, there is evidence to the contrary. One survey found that of 515 adult patients admitted to a poison treatment center for overdose, 26% of the men and 20% of the women could not be diagnosed as having psychiatric illness. Often, alcoholics have taken overdoses of barbiturates after drinking heavily. In fact the above survey pointed out that 56% of the men and 8% of the women were alcoholics. Moreover, 56% of the men and 23% of the women had been drinking just before they took the overdose.

In general, it is a moment of acute distress that prompts deliberate overdosing, regardless of the drug involved. The victim may have previously thought about doing so and may

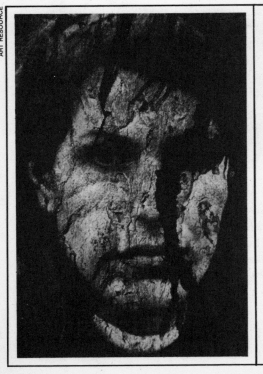

ART RESOURCE

This artist's rendering of a woman's face decomposing can be looked upon as an illustration of the feelings of desperation and hopelessness that often accompany drug abuse. Barbiturate overdose has sometimes occurred among alcoholics who, when intoxicated, have taken potentially lethal amounts of the drug without realizing it.

have even mentioned it to a friend. Unfortunately, such danger signals often go unheeded. Then the person is involved in a violent quarrel or experiences some severe emotional distress. Feeling hopeless, he or she acts irrationally and impulsively, and seeks escape.

The following is a typical case from the records of a poison control center:

> A 30-year-old woman, who had long endured an unhappy marriage to an aggressive ne'er-do-well, related how one day they had a protracted quarrel. There was violence, and she collapsed, crying, in an armchair. What was she to do? While she was weeping she remembered that a little while earlier a bottle of sleeping tablets had slipped down the back of the chair and she had never retrieved it. She reached down her hand, found the bottle, and took twenty Seconal capsules.

Those who abuse barbiturates range from young teenagers to habitual drug addicts. Actually, as we have already mentioned, relatively few teenagers do so. One study showed that of a sample of 80 teenagers who had used illicit drugs, only 10% regularly used barbiturates. Those who did used capsules of secobarbital or pentobarbital, or a mixture of secobarbital and amobarbital. They said they used the drugs both to escape from reality and to shock their parents. In fact, they said that they had used so much of the drug that they could not remember the actual experience.

In a 1980 New York State survey of 1,325 young adults, only 10% had ever used nonprescribed sedatives, including barbiturates, by age 18. By contrast, 79% had used marijuana and 30% had used cocaine. But by age 25, 19% had used nonprescribed barbiturates. More males (23%) than females (15%) had used illicit sedatives even though the difference was small in the number of males (9%) to females (6%) who had the drugs legally prescribed for them. In this group, those who first used the drugs between the ages of 14 and 20 were most likely to have obtained them illegally. Those who first started using them between the ages of 20 and 25 were most likely to have had their first contact through prescriptions. The New York study also reported that adolescent marijuana users were more likely than nonusers to start using other illicit drugs.

Abuse Among Professionals

Although drug abuse is most likely to catch the public's attention when it involves big-name athletes and entertainers, it is by now common knowledge that drug abuse also occurs among doctors, lawyers, and other professionals in high-status, high-stress jobs. To be sure, cocaine, stimulants, and marijuana are most often the drugs of choice among these types, but there is a significant incidence of barbiturate abuse as well. Often barbiturates are used in combination with stimulants in a frequently desperate effort on the part of the abuser to manage mood swings from euphoria to depression induced by each drug.

One dramatic case involved a 32-year-old pharmacist who suffered a grand mal seizure in the hospital parking lot. He was taken to the emergency room, and treated with short-

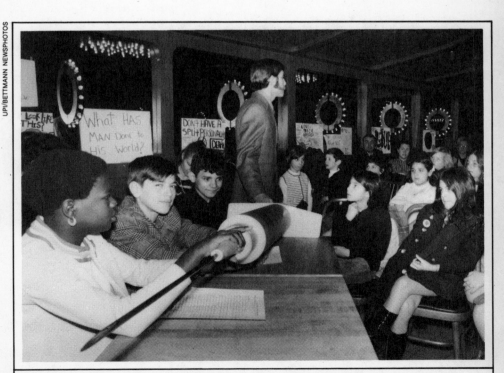

Children undergoing treatment for drug addiction at New York City's Phoenix House. Barbiturate abuse is relatively uncommon among teenagers, who tend most frequently to abuse alcohol and marijuana.

acting barbiturates. Based on his answers to interrogation by police and representatives of the American Pharmaceutical Association, it was determined that he had been taking approximately 30 to 40 Seconal capsules per day. His seizure resulted from the fact that he was being forced to cut back on his intake because his supply was drying up.

Using hospital stationery the pharmacist had been ordering secobarbital in large quantities from wholesale drug catalogues. When Seconal was delivered to the hospital pharmacy, he would steal several hundred capsules at a time. He would then purchase standard, unmarked red gelatin capsules and repackage the stolen Seconal, putting approximately 50

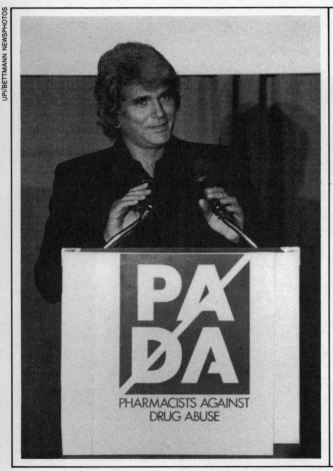

UPI/BETTMANN NEWSPHOTOS

Michael Landon makes an anti-drug speech at the annual meeting of the National Association of Chain Drug Stores. According to one study, barbiturate abusers who started taking these drugs between the ages of 20 and 25 were most likely to have had their first exposure through legal prescriptions.

mg (milligrams; 1 milligram is equal to .0035 ounces) in each capsule and keeping the remaining 50 mg for himself. He would then sell the unmarked capsules on the street as "reds" containing 100 mg of secobarbital. Because these capsules were unmarked, and all domestically manufactured drugs are marked with the drug company's logo, both law enforcement officials and the manufacturer erroneously assumed that the drug had been produced outside the United States.

As a result of these complex machinations, the pharmacist was able to generate substantial extra income as well as support his escalating barbiturate habit. As his thefts became larger, however, the hospital administration began to suspect that the thefts were occurring on the premises. But the man had avoided detection for two years, and there is no telling how long it would have taken the police to discover his illegal activities had his seizure not focused attention on him.

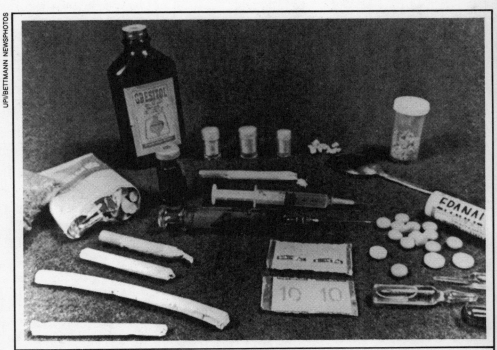

Because abuse of such drugs as marijuana, amphetamines, and barbiturates is now common among America's professional classes, many businesses have instituted measures to stamp out drug use in the workplace.

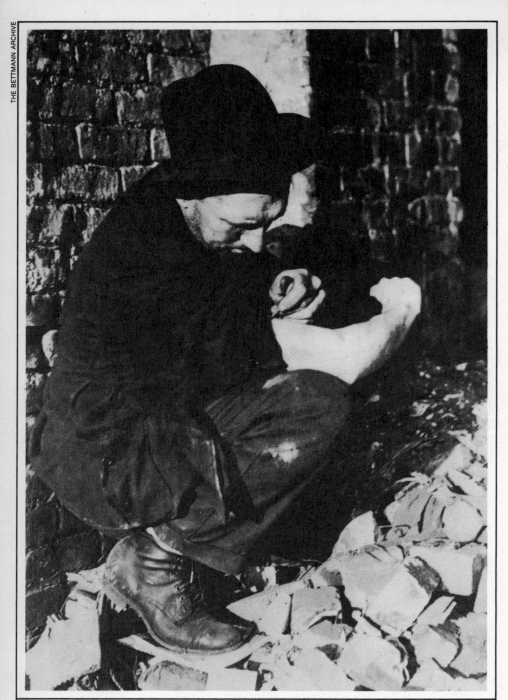

From the street substance this man is injecting to prescribed barbiturates, detecting any drug in the body of an overdose victim is a complicated but essential procedure.

CHAPTER 7

BARBITURATE OVERDOSE

For various clinical reasons, it is important to be able to detect barbiturates in the body. There are several highly complicated ways of doing this. Each drug is different and must be looked for separately. While some drugs are harder to detect than others, there are some characteristics shared by all barbiturates.

The first difficulty in testing for drugs involves the minuscule amounts of chemical being looked for. Finding a needle in a haystack may seem easy by comparison.

The second problem is that most drugs do not remain in their original states for long. The user's body quickly detoxifies the drug with enzymes, largely concentrated in the liver. The detoxification process changes the physical chemistry of the drug. It might consist, for example, of splitting the biologically active drug molecule into two inert pieces. Since they are produced by the body's metabolism of the drug, such pieces are called metabolites, whether the resulting pieces are inert, or just changed in their action. Oxygen and hydrogen atoms might be added to or taken away from the drug molecule, and even the slightest alteration in the chemical structure of barbiturates changes their properties radically.

The third problem in testing for drugs in the body is simply the great range of differences among them, in how they are made, and in what they do. Each one requires its own special test.

Despite these problems, there are factors that generally make drug detection possible. The first of these is that drugs, whether abused or taken properly, reach their target area, the central nervous system, through the blood. The drugs are mixed into the blood in a relatively even manner. Therefore, finding evidence of a drug in a small sample is a good indication of drug taking.

The second helpful factor is the way in which a drug leaves the body. It may leave in feces or urine. It may appear in saliva. It may be deposited in such tissues as skin, hair, and fingernails. Many drugs can be detected by examination of any of these biological samples. Some drugs are easier to detect than others but each drug leaves some telltale trail.

Finally, the ways in which drugs take effect are generally orderly. The amount of drug found in any particular biological sample is generally proportionate to the amount of drug actually taken and to the time that has elapsed since the drug was taken. In turn this means that most drug detection methods are not "all-or-none." Rather, a cut-off point can be set high enough so that a drug-positive result is obtained only if the drug was taken recently and in enough quantity to affect the person being tested. On the other hand, it should not be set so low that significant drug use would be missed.

For laboratory studies, in which a high degree of accuracy is required, three different systems are used. These are thin layer chromatography (TLC), gas-liquid chromatography (GLC), and gas chromatography/mass spectrometry (GC/MS). All are very accurate at identifying the type and quantity of drug present. They provide a sort of "fingerprint" for the drug which is then compared to the "fingerprints" produced by other substances.

The disadvantages of these systems lie in the fact that they are expensive, difficult to use and maintain, and require a highly trained staff to operate.

A more common instrument in drug abuse clinics and similar agencies is the Emit system. It is easy to set up and can be run by people with little technical training. It detects drugs in urine samples. The sample is mixed with substances containing bacteria, antibodies, and enzymes. Any drug present in the urine will reduce the activity of the enzymes.

The system is not as accurate as the GC/MS in determining the quantity of drug taken. But a moderate dose of a short-acting barbiturate can generally be detected for up to approximately 24 hours after ingestion. Longer-acting barbiturates such as phenobarbital can be detected for up to two to three weeks.

Treating Abuse and Overdose

Over the years since barbiturates became widely used in clinical medicine, various methods have been developed to treat the abuse of these drugs. Since barbiturates kill by depressing the respiratory system, the first objective in treating an overdose victim is simply to keep the person breathing. Treatment for overdose has become so advanced that someone who is hospitalized within 24 hours of taking an overdose is very likely to be saved. The exceptions are those overdose victims who have suffered irreversible heart, nerve, or kidney damage before treatment could be started.

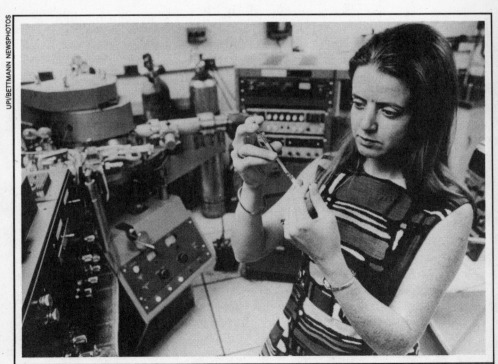

Highly sophisticated equipment like this gas mass spectrometer aids both hospital personnel and law enforcement officials in detecting and analyzing a wide variety of illicit drugs.

In the early 1950s a Danish physician, Dr. Carl Clemmesen, revolutionized the treatment of overdose victims. He established a poison treatment center and outlined a set of radically different procedures for treating barbiturate poisoning cases.

Between 1930 and 1950, the favored method of treatment had been to pump out the stomach and administer compounds that were thought to be antidotes for barbiturates. These were central nervous system stimulants such as pentylenetetrazol, nikethamide, and picrotoxin. These drugs stimulated breathing and became popular because in cases of mild overdose patients would wake up immediately after they were injected. In comatose patients, signs of stimulation would be seen, but relapse into coma invariably followed. Repeating doses of the stimulants in an effort to overcome the effects of the barbiturate could lead to exhaustion of the patient. In fact, in some cases such treatment would even worsen the shock produced by the barbiturate without speeding up recovery. In addition, these drugs disrupted the normal heart rate and caused convulsions. Finally, it was recognized that the effect of these antidotes was short-lived and often dangerous to the patient.

Dr. Clemmesen's procedures, known as the Scandinavian method, specifically advised against stomach pumping and the use of stimulants. Instead his method concentrated on two main areas. First, he used anesthesiological methods to keep the breathing lanes open and to provide continuous ventilation. Respirators could be used in the hospital, but in the field he advocated use of cardiopulmonary resuscitation, or CPR. Second, he urged close medical monitoring to combat shock by maintaining a stable body temperature, a balance in body fluids, and regular suction of the body's airways. Even prevention of bedsores was considered important.

Dr. Clemmesen rejected stomach pumping because of the possible damage it could cause to the lungs and bronchia. However, today's improved techniques now permit stomach pumping in hospitals, most often in cases where a drug has been taken within four hours of hospitalization.

In addition, treatment in very severe cases of barbiturate poisoning now includes forced administration of water and alkaline substances to encourage the body to excrete fluids. This speeds up the normal process of eliminating the drug from the body—especially in the case of phenobarbital. These procedures are generally used when it is expected that the coma induced will last at least 72 hours. This is especially vital when elderly patients are involved, because prolonged coma in such cases is often especially dangerous. The treatment can reduce the length of the coma by as much as 50%.

At first there was a great deal of controversy over use of the Scandinavian method in the United States, particularly over its rejection of the use of stimulants. However, it soon became apparent that the rate of survival from barbiturate overdose increased when treatment was based on Dr. Clemmesen's method.

A victim of drug abuse in New York City's Times Square area. Barbiturates depress the respiratory system in cases of severe overdose, a condition that, if left untreated, will result in death.

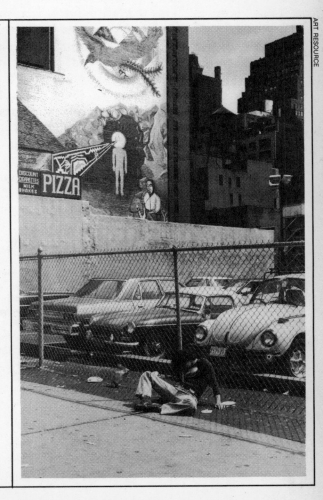

ART RESOURCE

One survey on the Scandinavian system's effectiveness reported that when steps were taken to maintain clear breathing, deaths from barbiturate overdose decreased from 25% of the cases to 15%. When special poison treatment centers began to be established, deaths further decreased to about 10% of the cases. When the use of central nervous system stimulants was discontinued, deaths decreased to 5%. The addition of modern therapy methods has reduced the death rate to less than 1%.

Getting Psychiatric Help

To be sure, some cases of barbiturate poisoning are the result of complications that arise during anesthesia and other medical treatments. However, some treatment centers report that up to 95% of people suffering from barbiturate poisoning took the overdose deliberately. Most such patients require psychiatric care and a small percentage are diagnosed as being mentally ill.

Doctors agree that anyone who has overdosed deliberately should be evaluated psychologically before being discharged. It does not matter how long the patient was in a coma or how seriously the patient's life was jeopardized.

For example, doctors say that someone who takes an overdose in front of family members with whom he or she is quarreling needs evaluation and treatment just as much as someone who takes an overdose in secret. Of course, not everyone who deliberately takes an overdose is mentally ill.

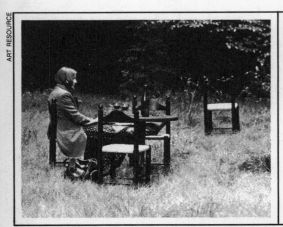

ART RESOURCE

One very serious danger with victims of deliberate barbiturate overdose is the possibility that they will attempt suicide again. This is particularly true among alcoholics and people suffering from clinical depression.

But certainly such a person is reacting in an extreme and violent manner to a moment of intense distress. A number of such people attempting suicide (we use the term "suicide" whether the victim truly seeks death or is making "a cry for help") will take a deliberate overdose again shortly after the first attempt. This is especially true in the case of alcoholics, those with personality problems, and housewives whose depression results from intolerable marriages.

A psychologist or psychiatrist evaluating a barbiturate overdose victim will attempt to develop a complete picture of the victim's situation: the circumstances immediately leading up to the victim's act; the sorts of conflicts and pressures that might have precipitated it; and his present and past psychiatric history. In addition, the mental health professional will make a particular effort to question someone close to the patient, a friend or relative. At the same time, the expert will have to be alert to the possibility that either or both the victim and the friend may wish to cover up or minimize certain aspects of the case.

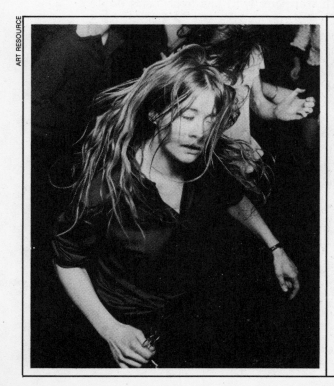

ART RESOURCE

Heavy use of barbiturates can eventually result in a disorientation that mimics psychosis. Overdoses are not always accidental; some treatment centers report that up to 95% of people suffering from barbiturate poisoning took the overdose deliberately.

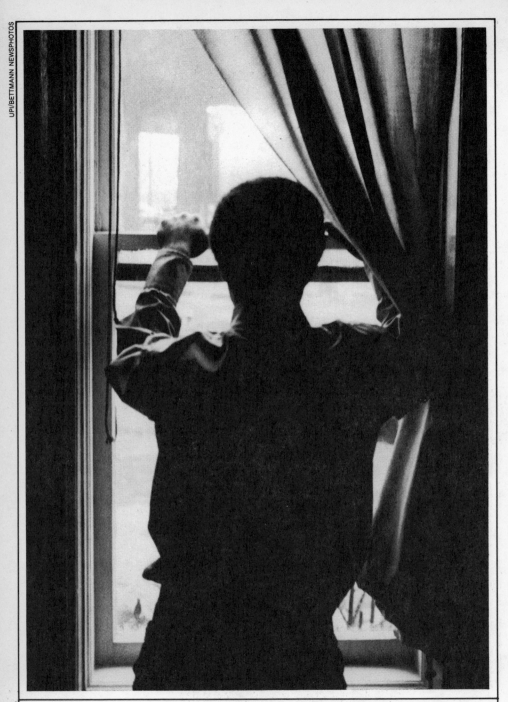

A patient at Odyssey House, a center for drug abusers in New York City. Barbiturates are indeed a double-edged sword, with both a high potential for abuse and an important role to play in clinical medicine.

CHAPTER 8

CONCLUSION

*I*n the decades since Fischer and von Mering synthesized the first barbiturates, the drugs themselves and the ways in which they are administered in clinical medicine have undergone many alterations and refinements. Experiments on both human and animal subjects have greatly advanced our knowledge of the ways in which the drugs work chemically and of the exact effects they have on the brain.

Although there was a time, climaxing in the 1950s and 1960s, when barbiturate abuse was rampant in American society, the days of widespread barbiturate abuse seem to be behind us. However, the barbiturates do have a high potential for abuse, physical dependence, and overdose that must not be underestimated. As a result, their use in the treatment of anxiety has been supplanted by the benzodiazepines, the family of drugs that includes the minor tranquilizers Librium and Valium. By the same token, the use of barbiturates as "sleeping pills" has been drastically reduced because of the danger that tolerance of the drug will lead to ever-increasing dosages that only achieve ever-diminishing results.

Thus, barbiturates are no longer widely used in treating the two maladies they were originally designed to alleviate—namely, anxiety and insomnia. Still, they continue to play an invaluable role in modern medicine. Properly administered, they are safe and sophisticated anesthetics, and their anticonvulsant properties make them the drugs of choice in treating epileptic and other seizures. With the increasingly advanced methods available for counteracting barbiturate overdose—whether inadvertent or intentional—the overall safety of barbiturate drug therapy has also been enhanced.

On balance, barbiturates hold a key position in the beneficial spectrum of modern pharmacology. However, they are powerful medicine indeed, and should only be taken and administered with the greatest possible caution.

APPENDIX 1

STREET TERMS RELATED TO BARBITURATES

STREET TERMS	TRADE NAME AND OR DESCRIPTION
abbotts	Nembutal (sodium pentobarbital) capsules
backwards	tranquilizers or barbiturates; to become rehabituated to a drug, to relapse
barb freak	intravenous barbiturate user
blockbusters	barbiturates; Nembutal (sodium pentobarbital) capsules
blue angels, bluebirds, blue bullets, blue devils, blue dolls, blue heavens, blues	amobarbital or Amytal capsules
candy	barbiturates; any drug a user likes
Christmas trees	Dexamyl (dextroamphetamine sulfate and amobarbital)
dolls	barbiturates
double trouble	capsules containing sodium secobarbital and sodium amobarbital; Tuinal; also generic products
down	barbiturates or any sedative drug; also a depressed state, sometimes related to intoxication but also to the absence of drugs
F-40s	Seconal (sodium secobarbital) capsules
G.B.s	barbiturates; goofballs
geronimo	alcohol mixed with barbiturates
goofballs	barbiturates
goofers	barbiturates; Doriden (glutethimide)
gorilla pills	capsules containing sodium secobarbital and sodium amobarbital; Tuinal; available as generic products
hearts	amphetamines; Dexamyl (dextroamphetamine sulfate and amobarbital) tablets
idiot pills	barbiturates
King Kong pills	barbiturates
Mexican reds	any red capsule containing Seconal (sodium secobarbital)
mother's little helper	Miltown, Equanil (meprobamate)
nebbies, nembies, nemmies	Nembutal (sodium pentobarbital) capsules
peanuts	barbiturates
phennies	phenobarbital tablets
pillhead	habitual user of barbiturates or amphetamines
pink ladies	barbiturates
pinks	any pinkish capsule containing sodium secobarbital; Seconal
purple hearts	Dexamyl (dextroamphetamine sulfate and amobarbital)
rainbows	see gorilla pills
R.D.s, reds, red birds, red bullets, red devils, red dolls	any red capsule containing sodium secobarbital; Seconal
reds and blues	see gorilla pills
seccies, seggies	Seconal (sodium secobarbital) capsules
sleepers, softballs, stumblers	downers, barbiturates, any central nervous system depressant
tootsies, trees, tuies	Tuinal (sodium secobarbital and sodium amobarbital)
wallbanger	someone showing lack of muscular coordination caused by intoxication with sedative-hypnotics or alcohol
yellow bullets, yellow dolls, yellow jackets, yellows	any yellow capsule containing pentobarbital; Nembutal

APPENDIX 2

STATE AGENCIES FOR THE PREVENTION AND TREATMENT OF DRUG ABUSE

ALABAMA
Department of Mental Health
Division of Mental Illness and
  Substance Abuse Community
  Programs
200 Interstate Park Drive
P.O. Box 3710
Montgomery, AL 36193
(205) 271-9253

ALASKA
Department of Health and Social
  Services
Office of Alcoholism and Drug
  Abuse
Pouch H-05-F
Juneau, AK 99811
(907) 586-6201

ARIZONA
Department of Health Services
Division of Behavioral Health
  Services
Bureau of Community Services
Alcohol Abuse and Alcoholism
  Section
2500 East Van Buren
Phoenix, AZ 85008
(602) 255-1238

Department of Health Services
Division of Behavioral Health
  Services
Bureau of Community Services
Drug Abuse Section
2500 East Van Buren
Phoenix, AZ 85008
(602) 255-1240

ARKANSAS
Department of Human Services
Office on Alcohol and Drug Abuse
  Prevention
1515 West 7th Avenue
Suite 310
Little Rock, AR 72202
(501) 371-2603

CALIFORNIA
Department of Alcohol and Drug
  Abuse
111 Capitol Mall
Sacramento, CA 95814
(916) 445-1940

COLORADO
Department of Health
Alcohol and Drug Abuse Division
4210 East 11th Avenue
Denver, CO 80220
(303) 320-6137

CONNECTICUT
Alcohol and Drug Abuse
  Commission
999 Asylum Avenue
3rd Floor
Hartford, CT 06105
(203) 566-4145

DELAWARE
Division of Mental Health
Bureau of Alcoholism and Drug
  Abuse
1901 North Dupont Highway
Newcastle, DE 19720
(302) 421-6101

DISTRICT OF COLUMBIA
Department of Human Services
Office of Health Planning and
  Development
601 Indiana Avenue, NW
Suite 500
Washington, D.C. 20004
(202) 724-5641

FLORIDA
Department of Health and
  Rehabilitative Services
Alcoholic Rehabilitation Program
1317 Winewood Boulevard
Room 187A
Tallahassee, FL 32301
(904) 488-0396

Department of Health and
  Rehabilitative Services
Drug Abuse Program
1317 Winewood Boulevard
Building 6, Room 155
Tallahassee, FL 32301
(904) 488-0900

GEORGIA
Department of Human Resources
Division of Mental Health and
  Mental Retardation
Alcohol and Drug Section
618 Ponce De Leon Avenue, NE
Atlanta, GA 30365-2101
(404) 894-4785

HAWAII
Department of Health
Mental Health Division
Alcohol and Drug Abuse Branch
1250 Punch Bowl Street
P.O. Box 3378
Honolulu, HI 96801
(808) 548-4280

IDAHO
Department of Health and Welfare
Bureau of Preventive Medicine
Substance Abuse Section
450 West State
Boise, ID 83720
(208) 334-4368

ILLINOIS
Department of Mental Health and
  Developmental Disabilities
Division of Alcoholism
160 North La Salle Street
Room 1500
Chicago, IL 60601
(312) 793-2907

Illinois Dangerous Drugs
  Commission
300 North State Street
Suite 1500
Chicago, IL 60610
(312) 822-9860

INDIANA
Department of Mental Health
Division of Addiction Services
429 North Pennsylvania Street
Indianapolis, IN 46204
(317) 232-7816

IOWA
Department of Substance Abuse
505 5th Avenue
Insurance Exchange Building
Suite 202
Des Moines, IA 50319
(515) 281-3641

KANSAS
Department of Social Rehabilitation
Alcohol and Drug Abuse Services
2700 West 6th Street
Biddle Building
Topeka, KS 66606
(913) 296-3925

KENTUCKY
Cabinet for Human Resources
Department of Health Services
Substance Abuse Branch
275 East Main Street
Frankfort, KY 40601
(502) 564-2880

LOUISIANA
Department of Health and Human
   Resources
Office of Mental Health and
   Substance Abuse
655 North 5th Street
P.O. Box 4049
Baton Rouge, LA 70821
(504) 342-2565

MAINE
Department of Human Services
Office of Alcoholism and Drug
   Abuse Prevention
Bureau of Rehabilitation
32 Winthrop Street
Augusta, ME 04330
(207) 289-2781

MARYLAND
Alcoholism Control Administration
201 West Preston Street
Fourth Floor
Baltimore, MD 21201
(301) 383-2977

State Health Department
Drug Abuse Administration
201 West Preston Street
Baltimore, MD 21201
(301) 383-3312

MASSACHUSETTS
Department of Public Health
Division of Alcoholism
755 Boylston Street
Sixth Floor
Boston, MA 02116
(617) 727-1960

Department of Public Health
Division of Drug Rehabilitation
600 Washington Street
Boston, MA 02114
(617) 727-8617

MICHIGAN
Department of Public Health
Office of Substance Abuse Services
3500 North Logan Street
P.O. Box 30035
Lansing, MI 48909
(517) 373-8603

MINNESOTA
Department of Public Welfare
Chemical Dependency Program
   Division
Centennial Building
658 Cedar Street
4th Floor
Saint Paul, MN 55155
(612) 296-4614

MISSISSIPPI
Department of Mental Health
Division of Alcohol and Drug Abuse
1102 Robert E. Lee Building
Jackson, MS 39201
(601) 359-1297

MISSOURI
Department of Mental Health
Division of Alcoholism and Drug
   Abuse
2002 Missouri Boulevard
P.O. Box 687
Jefferson City, MO 65102
(314) 751-4942

MONTANA
Department of Institutions
Alcohol and Drug Abuse Division
1539 11th Avenue
Helena, MT 59620
(406) 449-2827

NEBRASKA
Department of Public Institutions
Division of Alcoholism and Drug Abuse
801 West Van Dorn Street
P.O. Box 94728
Lincoln, NB 68509
(402) 471-2851, Ext. 415

NEVADA
Department of Human Resources
Bureau of Alcohol and Drug Abuse
505 East King Street
Carson City, NV 89710
(702) 885-4790

NEW HAMPSHIRE
Department of Health and Welfare
Office of Alcohol and Drug Abuse
   Prevention
Hazen Drive
Health and Welfare Building
Concord, NH 03301
(603) 271-4627

NEW JERSEY
Department of Health
Division of Alcoholism
129 East Hanover Street CN 362
Trenton, NJ 08625
(609) 292-8949

Department of Health
Division of Narcotic and Drug Abuse
   Control
129 East Hanover Street CN 362
Trenton, NJ 08625
(609) 292-8949

NEW MEXICO
Health and Environment Department
Behavioral Services Division
Substance Abuse Bureau
725 Saint Michaels Drive
P.O. Box 968
Santa Fe, NM 87503
(505) 984-0020, Ext. 304

NEW YORK
Division of Alcoholism and Alcohol
   Abuse
194 Washington Avenue
Albany, NY 12210
(518) 474-5417

Division of Substance Abuse
   Services
Executive Park South
Box 8200
Albany, NY 12203
(518) 457-7629

NORTH CAROLINA
Department of Human Resources
Division of Mental Health, Mental
   Retardation and Substance Abuse
   Services
Alcohol and Drug Abuse Services
325 North Salisbury Street
Albemarle Building
Raleigh, NC 27611
(919) 733-4670

NORTH DAKOTA
Department of Human Services
Division of Alcoholism and Drug
   Abuse
State Capitol Building
Bismarck, ND 58505
(701) 224-2767

OHIO
Department of Health
Division of Alcoholism
246 North High Street
P.O. Box 118
Columbus, OH 43216
(614) 466-3543

Department of Mental Health
Bureau of Drug Abuse
65 South Front Street
Columbus, OH 43215
(614) 466-9023

OKLAHOMA
Department of Mental Health
Alcohol and Drug Programs
4545 North Lincoln Boulevard
Suite 100 East Terrace
P.O. Box 53277
Oklahoma City, OK 73152
(405) 521-0044

OREGON
Department of Human Resources
Mental Health Division
Office of Programs for Alcohol and
Drug Problems
2575 Bittern Street, NE
Salem, OR 97310
(503) 378-2163

PENNSYLVANIA
Department of Health
Office of Drug and Alcohol
Programs
Commonwealth and Forster Avenues
Health and Welfare Building
P.O. Box 90
Harrisburg, PA 17108
(717) 787-9857

RHODE ISLAND
Department of Mental Health,
Mental Retardation and Hospitals
Division of Substance Abuse
Substance Abuse Administration
Building
Cranston, RI 02920
(401) 464-2091

SOUTH CAROLINA
Commission on Alcohol and Drug
Abuse
3700 Forest Drive
Columbia, SC 29204
(803) 758-2521

SOUTH DAKOTA
Department of Health
Division of Alcohol and Drug Abuse
523 East Capitol, Joe Foss Building
Pierre, SD 57501
(605) 773-4806

TENNESSEE
Department of Mental Health and
Mental Retardation
Alcohol and Drug Abuse Services
505 Deaderick Street
James K. Polk Building, Fourth Floor
Nashville, TN 37219
(615) 741-1921

TEXAS
Commission on Alcoholism
809 Sam Houston State Office Building
Austin, TX 78701
(512) 475-2577

Department of Community Affairs
Drug Abuse Prevention Division
2015 South Interstate Highway 35
P.O. Box 13166
Austin, TX 78711
(512) 443-4100

UTAH
Department of Social Services
Division of Alcoholism and Drugs
150 West North Temple
Suite 350
P.O. Box 2500
Salt Lake City, UT 84110
(801) 533-6532

VERMONT
Agency of Human Services
Department of Social and
Rehabilitation Services
Alcohol and Drug Abuse Division
103 South Main Street
Waterbury, VT 05676
(802) 241-2170

VIRGINIA
Department of Mental Health and
Mental Retardation
Division of Substance Abuse
109 Governor Street
P.O. Box 1797
Richmond, VA 23214
(804) 786-5313

WASHINGTON
Department of Social and Health
Service
Bureau of Alcohol and Substance
Abuse
Office Building—44 W
Olympia, WA 98504
(206) 753-5866

WEST VIRGINIA
Department of Health
Office of Behavioral Health Services
Division on Alcoholism and Drug
Abuse
1800 Washington Street East
Building 3 Room 451
Charleston, WV 25305
(304) 348-2276

WISCONSIN
Department of Health and Social
Services
Division of Community Services
Bureau of Community Programs
Alcohol and Other Drug Abuse
Program Office
1 West Wilson Street
P.O. Box 7851
Madison, WI 53707
(608) 266-2717

WYOMING
Alcohol and Drug Abuse Programs
Hathaway Building
Cheyenne, WY 82002
(307) 777-7115, Ext. 7118

GUAM
Mental Health & Substance Abuse
Agency
P.O. Box 20999
Guam 96921

PUERTO RICO
Department of Addiction Control
Services
Alcohol Abuse Programs
P.O. Box B-Y Rio Piedras Station
Rio Piedras, PR 00928
(809) 763-5014

Department of Addiction Control
Services
Drug Abuse Programs
P.O. Box B-Y Rio Piedras Station
Rio Piedras, PR 00928
(809) 764-8140

VIRGIN ISLANDS
Division of Mental Health,
Alcoholism & Drug Dependency
Services
P.O. Box 7329
Saint Thomas, Virgin Islands 00801
(809) 774-7265

AMERICAN SAMOA
LBJ Tropical Medical Center
Department of Mental Health Clinic
Pago Pago, American Samoa 96799

TRUST TERRITORIES
Director of Health Services
Office of the High Commissioner
Saipan, Trust Territories 96950

anorexia   prolonged loss of appetite

antispasmodic   capable of preventing or relieving spasms or convulsions

barbiturate   a drug that causes depression of the central nervous system; generally used to reduce anxiety or to induce euphoria

barbituric acid   a chemical, derived from pyrimidine, which forms the basis for barbiturates

benzodiazepines   depressants that are potent relievers of anxiety and insomnia

bromides   compounds based on the element bromine that are used as sedatives

bronchial tree   the main branches and smaller tubes of the bronchi that serve as air passageways from the trachea to the lungs

catatonic schizophrenia   a mental disorder in which patients remain mute and stay in fixed positions for a long time

depressant   a drug that slows the activity of the central nervous system

electroencephalogram   the record of brain waves used to detect abnormal brain activity

Emit system   an instrument that detects traces of drugs in urine samples

hyperthermia   extremely high fever

hypnotic   a sleep-inducing agent

intermediate-acting drug   a drug having effects that last between 4 and 6 hours

long-acting drug   a drug having effects that last for 6 hours or more

metabolism   the chemical changes in the living cell by which energy is provided for the vital body processes and activities and by which new material is assimilated to repair cell structures; or, the process that uses enzymes to convert one substance into compounds that can be easily eliminated from the body

narcotic   originally, a group of drugs producing effects similar to morphine; often used to refer to any substance that sedates, has a depressive effect, and/or causes dependence

necrosis   severe tissue damage that occurs when a drug is injected into an artery rather than a vein

neuron   the fundamental unit of nerve tissue

neurotransmitter   a chemical that travels from the axon of one neuron, across the synaptic gap, and to the receptor site on the dendrite of an adjacent neuron, thus allowing communication between neural cells

opiate   a compound from the milky juice of the poppy plant *Papaver somniferum*, including opium, morphine, codeine, and their derivatives, such as heroin

pharmacokinetics   study of the metabolism and action of drugs, how they are absorbed into, distributed throughout, and eliminated from the body

pharmacology   the study of the properties and reactions of drugs and how they affect the functioning of organisms

physical dependence   an adaptation of the body to the presence of a drug, such that its absence produces withdrawal symptoms

placebo   a substance that is pharmacologically inactive and is used as a control in experiments measuring the effectiveness of another substance, or is administered in order to satisfy the psychological needs of patients

porphyria   an ailment, often inherited, that is characterized by severe skin conditions such as extreme sensitivity to sunlight

psychological dependence   a condition in which the drug user craves a drug to maintain a sense of well-being and feels discomfort when deprived of it

Scandinavian method   a revolutionary treatment for overdose victims developed by Dr. Carl Clemmesen. The method called for using cardiopulmonary resuscitation and medical monitoring to maintain a steady body temperature

sedative   a drug that produces calmness, relaxation, and, at high doses, sleep; includes barbiturates

short-acting drug   a drug having effects that last for less than 4 hours

sleep therapy   a drug-induced sleep used for psychiatric treatment

synapse   the gap between the axon and dendrite of two adjacent neurons in which neurotransmitters travel

tolerance   a decrease of susceptibility to the effects of a drug due to its continued administration, resulting in the user's need to increase the drug dosage in order to achieve the effects experienced previously

trauma   a condition of severe shock following a physical or emotional blow

ultra-short-acting drug   drugs that are usually given by injection and that may produce sedation before the injection is complete

withdrawal   the physiological and psychological effects that occur after the use of a drug is discontinued

Further Reading

Brecher, E.M., and the Editors of *Consumer Reports*. *Licit and Illicit Drugs.* Boston: Little, Brown and Co., 1972.

Gilman, A.G., Goodman, L.S., and Gilman, A. *The Pharmacological Basis of Therapeutics.* New York: MacMillan Publishing Co., Inc., 1980.

Matthew, H. *Acute Barbiturate Poisoning.* Amsterdam: Excerpta Medica, 1971.

National Institute on Drug Abuse. *First Triennial Report to Congress on Drug Dependence Research*, chapter on sedatives and anti-anxiety agents. NIDA Research Monograph, Washington, D.C.: U.S. Government Printing Office, 1984.

Index

Nancy Ator, Ph.D., received her degree in behavioral pharmacology at the University of Maryland. She is an assistant professor of behavioral biology at The Johns Hopkins University School of Medicine. Dr. Ator is engaged in research on sedatives and tranquilizers.

Dr. Jack E. Henningfield received a Ph.D. in psychopharmacology from the University of Minnesota. He is an assistant professor of behavioral biology at The Johns Hopkins University School of Medicine. He is also chief of the Biology of Dependence and Abuse Potential Assessment Laboratory at the Addiction Research Center of the National Institute on Drug Abuse.

Solomon H. Snyder, M.D., is Distinguished Service Professor of Neuroscience, Pharmacology and Psychiatry at The Johns Hopkins University School of Medicine. He has served as president of the Society for Neuroscience and in 1978 received the Albert Laster Award in Medical Research. He has authored *Uses of Marijuana, Madness and the Brain, The Troubled Mind, Biological Aspects of Mental Disorder,* and edited *Perspective in Neuropharmacology: A Tribute to Julius Axelrod.* Professor Snyder was a research associate with Dr. Axelrod at the National Institutes of Health.

Barry L. Jacobs, Ph.D., is currently a professor in the program of neuroscience at Princeton University. Professor Jacobs is author of *Serotonin Neurotransmission and Behavior* and *Hallucinogens: Neurochemical, Behavioral and Clinical Perspectives.* He has written many journal articles in the field of neuroscience and contributed numerous chapters to books on behavior and brain science. He has been a member of several panels of the National Institute of Mental Health.

Jerome H. Jaffe, M.D., formerly professor of psychiatry at the College of Physicians and Surgeons, Columbia University, has been named recently Director of the Addiction Research Center of the National Institute on Drug Abuse. Dr. Jaffe is also a psychopharmacologist and has conducted research on a wide range of addictive drugs and developed treatment programs for addicts. He has acted as Special Consultant to the President on Narcotics and Dangerous Drugs and was the first director of the White House Special Action Office for Drug Abuse Prevention.